Preface iMIMI(

The second edition of the workshop on Interpretability of Machine Intelligence in Medical Image Computing (iMIMIC 2019)[1] was held on October 17, 2019, as a half day satellite event of the 22nd International Conference on Medical Image Computing and Computer Assisted Intervention (MICCAI 2019), in Shenzhen, China. With its second edition, this workshop aimed at introducing the challenges and opportunities of interpretability of machine learning systems in the context of MICCAI, as well as understanding the current state of the art in the topic and promoting it as a crucial area for further research. The workshop program comprised oral presentations of the accepted works and two keynotes provided by experts in the field.

Machine learning systems are achieving remarkable performances at the cost of increased complexity. Hence, they become less interpretable, which may cause distrust. As these systems are pervasively being introduced to critical domains, such as medical image computing and computer-assisted intervention, it becomes imperative to develop methodologies to explain their predictions. Such methodologies would help physicians to decide whether they should follow/trust a prediction. Additionally, it could facilitate the deployment of such systems, from a legal perspective. Ultimately, interpretability is closely related with AI safety in healthcare. Besides increasing trust and acceptance by physicians, interpretability of machine learning systems can be helpful for other purposes, such as during method development, for revealing biases in the training data, or for studying and identifying the most relevant data (e.g., specific MRI sequences in multi-sequence acquisitions).

The iMIMIC 2019 proceedings include seven papers of eight pages each, carefully selected from a larger pool of submitted manuscripts, following a rigorous single-blinded peer-review process. Each paper was reviewed by at least two expert reviewers. All the accepted papers were presented as oral presentations during the workshop, with time for questions and discussion.

We thank all the authors for their participation and the Technical Committee members for contributing to this workshop. We are also very grateful to our sponsors and supporters.

September 2019

Mauricio Reyes
Ender Konukoglu
Ben Glocker
Roland Wiest

The original version of the book was revised: the display of the volume editor's name on SpringerLink was fixed. The correction to the book is available at https://doi.org/10.1007/978-3-030-33850-3_11

---

[1] https://imimic-workshop.com/.

Organization

Organization Committee

Mauricio Reyes	University of Bern, Switzerland
Ender Konukoglu	ETHZ, Switzerland
Ben Glocker	Imperial College, UK
Roland Wiest	University Hospital of Bern, Switzerland

Technical Committee

Bjoern Menze	Technical University of Munich, Germany
Carlos A. Silva	University of Minho, Portugal
Dwarikanath Mahapatra	IBM Research, Australia
Nick Pawlowski	Imperial College London, UK
Hrvoje Bogunovic	Medical University of Vienna, Austria
Wilson Silva	University of Porto, Portugal
Islem Rekik	Istanbul Technical University, Turkey
Raphael Meier	University Hospital Bern, Switzerland
Sérgio Pereira	University of Minho, Portugal

Preface ML-CDS 2019

On behalf of the Organizing Committee, we welcome you to the 9th Workshop on Multimodal Learning for Clinical Decision Support (ML-CDS 2019). The goal of these series of workshops is to bring together researchers in medical imaging, medical image retrieval, data mining, text retrieval, and machine learning/AI communities to discuss new techniques of multimodal mining/retrieval and their use in clinical decision support. Although the title of the workshop has changed slightly over the years, the common theme preserved is the notion of clinical decision support and the need for multimodal analysis. The previous seven workshops on this topic have been well-received at MICCAI, specifically Granada (2018), Quebec City (2017), Athens (2016), Munich (2015), Nagoya (2013), Nice (2012), Toronto (2011), and London (2009).

Continuing on the momentum built by these workshops, our focus remains on multimodal learning. As has been the norm with these workshops, the papers were submitted in eight-page double-blind format and were accepted after review. The workshop continues to stay with an oral format for all the presentations. There was a lively panel composed of doctors, medical imaging researchers, and industry experts. This year we also invited researchers to participate in a tubes and lines detection challenge within the program.

With less than 5% of medical image analysis techniques translating to clinical practice, workshops on this topic have helped to raise awareness of our field to clinical practitioners. The approach taken in this workshop is to scale it to large collections of patient data exposing interesting issues of multimodal learning and its specific use in clinical decision support by practicing physicians. With the introduction of intelligent browsing and summarization methods, we hope to also address the ease of use in conveying derived information to clinicians to aid their adoption. Finally, the ultimate impact of these methods can be judged when they begin to affect treatment planning in clinical practice.

We hope that you enjoyed the program we assembled, and we thank you for your active participation in the discussion on the topics of the papers and the panel.

September 2019

Tanveer Syeda-Mahmood
Yaniv Gur
Hayit Greenspan
Anant Madabhushi

Organization

Program Chairs

Tanveer Syeda-Mahmood   IBM Research - Almaden, USA
Yaniv Gur   IBM Research - Almaden, USA
Hayit Greenspan   Tel-Aviv University, Israel
Anant Madabhushi   Case Western Reserve University, USA

Program Committee

Amir Amini   University of Louisville, USA
Sameer Antani   National Library of Medicine, USA
Rivka Colen   MD Andersen Research Center, USA
Keyvan Farahani   National Cancer Institute, USA
Alejandro Frangi   University of Sheffield, UK
Guido Gerig   New York University, USA
David Gutman   Emory University, USA
Allan Halpern   Memorial Sloan-Kettering Research Center, USA
Ghassan Hamarneh   Simon Fraser University, Canada
Jayshree Kalpathy-Kramer   Mass General Hospital, USA
Ron Kikinis   Harvard University, USA
Georg Langs   Medical University of Vienna, Austria
Robert Lundstrom   Kaiser Permanente, USA
B. Manjunath   University of California, Santa Barbara, USA
Dimitris Metaxas   Rutgers, USA
Nikos Paragios   École centrale de Paris, France
Daniel Racoceanu   Sorbonne University, France
Eduardo Romero   Universidad Nationale Colombia, Colombia
Daniel Rubin   Stanford University, USA
Russ Taylor   Johns Hopkins University, USA
Agma Traina   Sao Paulo University, Brazil
Max Viergewer   Utrecht University, The Netherlands
Sean Zhou   United Imaging Intelligence, Shanghai, China

Contents

Second International Workshop on Interpretability of Machine Intelligence in Medical Image Computing (iMIMIC 2019)

Testing the Robustness of Attribution Methods for Convolutional Neural Networks in MRI-Based Alzheimer's Disease Classification

Fabian Eitel[1,2,3], Kerstin Ritter[1,2,3(✉)],
and for the Alzheimer's Disease Neuroimaging Initiative (ADNI)

[1] Department of Psychiatry and Psychotherapy, Charité – Universitätsmedizin
Berlin, corporate member of Freie Universität Berlin, Humboldt-Universität zu Berlin,
and Berlin Institute of Health (BIH), 10117 Berlin, Germany
kerstin.ritter@charite.de
[2] Berlin Center for Advanced Neuroimaging, Charité – Universitätsmedizin Berlin,
corporate member of Freie Universität Berlin, Humboldt-Universität zu Berlin,
and Berlin Institute of Health (BIH), 10117 Berlin, Germany
[3] Bernstein Center for Computational Neuroscience,
10117 Berlin, Germany

Abstract. Attribution methods are an easy to use tool for investigating and validating machine learning models. Multiple methods have been suggested in the literature and it is not yet clear which method is most suitable for a given task. In this study, we tested the robustness of four attribution methods, namely gradient * input, guided backpropagation, layer-wise relevance propagation and occlusion, for the task of Alzheimer's disease classification. We have repeatedly trained a convolutional neural network (CNN) with identical training settings in order to separate structural MRI data of patients with Alzheimer's disease and healthy controls. Afterwards, we produced attribution maps for each subject in the test data and quantitatively compared them across models and attribution methods. We show that visual comparison is not sufficient and that some widely used attribution methods produce highly inconsistent outcomes.

Keywords: Machine learning · Convolutional neural networks · MRI · Explainability · Robustness · Attribution methods · Alzheimer's disease

1 Introduction

As machine learning becomes more and more abundant in medical imaging, it is necessary to validate its efficacy with the same standards as other techniques. On magnetic resonance imaging (MRI) data, several studies have reported classification accuracies above 90% when using machine learning to detect neurological and psychiatric diseases (for a review, see [17]). While these results seem

ⓒ Springer Nature Switzerland AG 2019
K. Suzuki et al. (Eds.): ML-CDS 2019/IMIMIC 2019, LNCS 11797, pp. 3–11, 2019.
https://doi.org/10.1007/978-3-030-33850-3_1

promising at first, an in-depth investigation of those results both in terms of generalizability as well as medical validity is necessary before they can enter clinical practice. Medical validity can be examined by using attribution methods such as saliency analysis. Specifically, the decision of a machine learning algorithm can be visualized as a heatmap in the image space, in which the contribution of each voxel is determined. To identify the relevance of specific brain areas, quantitative and qualitative analyses on the heatmaps can be performed. Models that shift importance to areas which are well known to be clinically relevant in specific diseases might be more suitable for clinical practice in comparison with models that scatter relevance across the entire image or to seemingly random brain areas. While it might not be necessary to understand the exact workings of a model, similar to many drugs used in clinical practice, the causal mechanism of a model should have at least a minimal coherence with the causal reasoning of a clinical expert and should be interpretable by the expert.

In neuroimaging studies, where sample sizes are often extremely limited, specific attention needs to be given to robustness. Small sample sizes can cause model training to be rather fluctuating and varying between different runs. One can avoid "cherry-picking" of final results easily by identically repeating training procedures and reporting average scores. In doing so, the question arises whether attribution methods suffer from similar variances. In the present study, we therefore propose to evaluate the *robustness* of attribution methods. Specifically, we investigate whether multiple heatmap methods are coherent in their results over identical training repetitions with a variety of measures. For this purpose, we trained a convolutional neural network (CNN) several times to separate structural MRI data of patients with Alzheimer's disease (AD) and healthy controls. For each subject in the test data, we then produced heatmaps using four widely used attribution methods, namely gradient * input, guided backpropagation, layer-wise relevance propagation (LRP) and occlusion. All those methods have been applied in MRI-based AD classification before [5,8,12]. As it was noted in [16] specific criteria are needed in order to avoid artifacts from the data, the model or the explanation method in order to empirically compare them. Here we point out the issue of artifacts from model training and present a framework to investigate them.

2   Related Work

Different criteria for evaluating visualization methods have been proposed in the literature, including sensitivity, implementation invariance, completeness and linearity [16], selectivity [3], conservation and positivity [10] as well as continuity [11]. Additionally, [1] has introduced two sanity checks of visualization methods based on network and data permutation tests. Only [2] has investigated robustness so far. We differ from [2] by repeating the training cycle and comparing the outcomes without any perturbation.

In neuroimaging, only a few studies have compared attribution methods. [12] has given an overview of four different attribution methods for MRI-based

Alzheimer's disease classification and introduced a modified version of occlusion, in which brain areas according to an atlas are occluded. For the same task, [5] has presented an in-depth analysis together with multiple metrics for evaluating attribution methods based on LRP and guided backpropagation as a baseline method. In [6], it has been shown that LRP and gradient * input led to almost identical results for MRI-based multiple sclerosis detection.

3 Methods

The dataset used in this study is part of the Alzheimer's Disease Neuroimaging Initiative[1] (ADNI) cohort. Specifically, we have collected 969 T1-weighted MPRAGE sequences from 344 participants (193 AD patients and 151 healthy controls) of up to three time-points. The full-sized 1 mm isotropic images were non-linearly registered using the ANTs framework to the ICBM152 (2009c) atlas. We have split the dataset patient-wise by sampling 30 participants from each class into a test set and 18 participants from each class into a validation set. All available time-points were then used to increase the total sample size. Additionally, the data was augmented by flipping along the sagittal axis with a probability of 50% and translated along the coronal axis between −2 and 2 voxels.

The 3D-CNN used to separate AD patients and healthy controls consists of 4 blocks of Conv-BatchNorm-ReLU-MaxPool followed by two fully-connected layers, the first being activated by a ReLU as well. A dropout of 0.4 was applied before each fully-connected layer. All convolutional layers use $3 \times 3 \times 3$ filters, with 8, 16, 31, 64 filters from bottom to top layers. Max pooling uses a pooling size of 2, 3, 2, 3 voxels respectively. We used the ADAM optimizer with an initial learning rate of 0.0001 and a weight decay of 0.0001. Furthermore, early stopping with a patience of 8 epochs was employed. The training was repeated for 10 times to create 10 identically trained models, albeit each randomly initialized. Note that mini-batch ordering was not fixed between different runs.

For each trained model and each subject in the test set, we produced heatmaps using the following attribution methods:

Gradient * input [13] multiplies the gradient, which has been backpropagated into the input space, with the original input. It is an adaption of saliency maps [14] and increases the sharpness of the resulting heatmaps.

Guided backpropagation [15] modifies the backpropagation in ReLU layers by only passing positive gradients. Since the backpropagation ignores features in which the ReLU activation is zero, guided backpropagation requires both the gradient and the activation to be non-zero.

Layer-wise relevance propagation (LRP) [3] backpropagates the classification score instead of the gradient and multiplies it with the normalized activation for each neuron. LRP conserves the relevance under certain conditions such that the sum of relevance for all neurons does not change between layers.

---

[1] http://adni.loni.usc.edu/.

Occlusion [18] is, unlike the other presented methods, not based on back-propagation. In occlusion, the attribution is computed by the change in the output score, when some part of the input example is "occluded" (i.e. set to zero). Here, we occlude a volumetric patch which is shifted over the entire MRI volume. Although the occlusion method results commonly in much coarser heatmaps (depending on the size of the patch), we included this method because it has been used several times in MRI-based AD classification [7–9,12].

Besides comparing the attribution maps directly, we have carried out atlas-based comparisons using the Neuromorphometrics atlas [4] in which left and right hemisphere regions have been combined. We computed the attribution within each region based on three metrics: **sum** as the sum of absolute values in each region, **density** as the regional mean, i.e. the sum normalized by the size of the respective region, as well as **gain** as the ratio between the sum for patients divided by the sum for healthy controls. The latter was defined in [5] arguing that healthy controls typically also receive positive relevance. By normalizing each region to a control average those regions which exhibit strong differences between controls and patients are highlighted. When sorting brain areas by these metrics, we therefore obtain three rankings for each repetition and method. We then compare the intersection between the top 10 regions of each repetition in order to see whether repeated runs highlight similar regions.

4   Results

The balanced accuracy of all 10 training runs on the test set is on average 86.74% with a considerable range of 83.06% to 90.12% between runs.

Figure 1 shows the guided backpropagation attribution maps, averaged over all true positives for each of the 10 training runs. Solely by visually inspecting them, one can see clear differences between the various runs. While some heatmaps seem to highlight the hippocampus (top row middle, bottom row 2nd to 4th) others do not (top row 1st and 4th, bottom row 5th). In almost all heatmaps the edges of the brain are given attribution and in some a large amounts are given to the cerebellum (bottom row 1st, 2nd and 5th). The heatmaps from the other methods exhibit similar variances.

Guided backpropagation heatmap averages for true positives

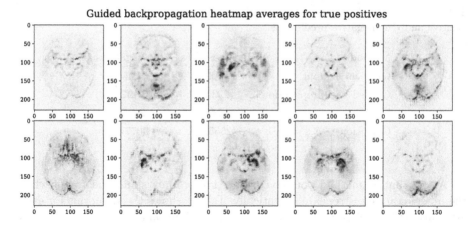

Fig. 1. Different heatmap outcomes (averaged over all true positives) for guided back-propagation and each of the 10 trained models.

In Fig. 2, we compare the four different attribution methods. Occlusion clearly stands out by producing a much coarser attribution map than the other methods. This is due to the fact that the size of the patch which is being occluded, scales inversely with the run-time. Running the occlusion method for a 3D image with a patch size of $1 \times 1 \times 1$, in order to match the sharpness of the other methods, would be computationally unfeasible. One can also note that gradient * input seems to produce the least continuous regions. With exception of occlusion, all methods seem to attribute importance to the hippocampus.

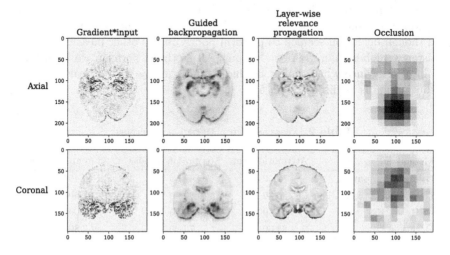

Fig. 2. Averages over all true positive attribution maps and all 10 runs for each attribution method.

Table 1. L2-norm between average attribution maps of all different runs for true positive and true negative predictions.

Method	True positives	True negatives
Gradient * input	3102	3145
Guided backpropagation	2930	**1992**
LRP	**2241**	2196
Occlusion	25553	30774

An attribution method would be expected to produce similar heatmaps when the model training is repeated identically. Table 1 shows the L2-norms for each attribution method, between all of its average attribution maps. LRP and guided backpropagation have the smallest L2-norms between their average heatmaps. Occlusion has L2-norms by a magnitude larger than the other methods, which might be due to the limited sharpness. Average heatmaps have been scaled by their maximum value to produce comparable results.

When dividing the attributions into brain regions, large regions such as cerebral white matter and the cerebellum receive most attribution. Normalized by region size, the basal forebrain, 4th ventricle, hippocampus and amygdala become highlighted. Standardizing by attributions of healthy controls leads to rather inconsistent orderings. In Fig. 3, we show how much the top 10 brain regions, in terms of attribution, intersect with each other over repetitions. An intersection of 100% means that the regions between those two runs contain the same regions in their top 10, ignoring the order within those 10. In Table 2, we averaged the intersections separately for each attribution method and each metric. All methods have their highest intersection in terms of region-wise sum, guided backpropgation and LRP seem to reproduce the same regions almost perfectly. Even though occlusion seemed to perform poorly in the other measures it has a consistency higher than gradient * input. All methods perform worst in terms of gain of relevance which might be due to the scarcity within healthy control attribution maps as discussed in [5].

Table 2. Averages of top 10 region coherence.

Method	Attribution sum	Attribution density	Gain of attribution
Gradient * input	72.60 %	69.00 %	46.40 %
Guided backpropagation	96.60 %	80.60 %	68.60 %
LRP	96.80 %	88.40 %	78.00 %
Occlusion	84.60 %	74.20 %	67.80 %

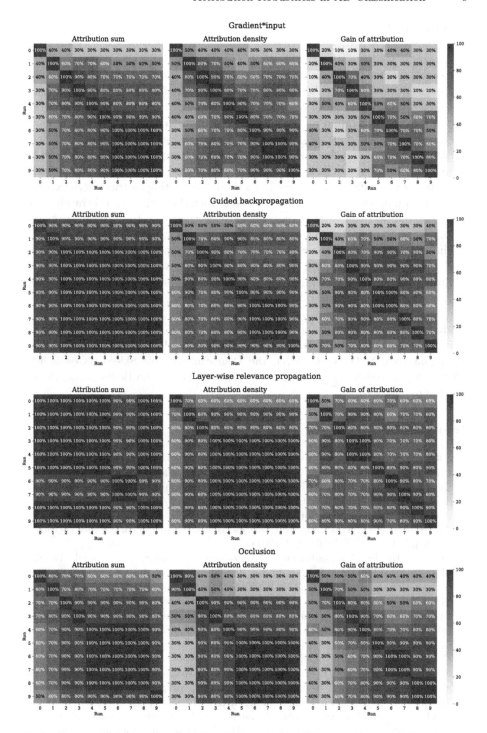

Fig. 3. Intersection between the 10 regions with the highest attribution according to the total sum, the size-normalized density and the control-normalized gain.

5   Discussion

In this study, we have shown that attribution methods differ in robustness with respect to repeated model training. In particular, we found that LRP and guided backpropagation produce the most coherent attribution maps, both in terms of distance between attribution maps as well as in terms of order of attribution awarded to individual regions. We also confirm that solely visually judging heatmaps is a deficient criteria as pointed out by [1]. Especially in medical imaging, it is important to acknowledge that the small sample sizes available lead to variances in the output. These variances make it hard to compare and to replicate outcomes of individual studies. Even though reporting metrics averaged over repeated training runs is an effective tool to reduce the variances, it is rarely used in the community. Here, we have extended the repetition to attribution methods and shown similar variances. Even though these variances likely stem from the different local minima each training run ended up in, attribution methods which cease the variances and report similar outcomes are highly preferable. In conclusion, we think that domain specific metrics, as suggested in this study, are essential for identifying suitable attribution methods.

Funding. We acknowledge support from the German Research Foundation (DFG, 389563835), the Manfred and Ursula-Müller Stiftung, the Brain & Behavior Research Foundation (NARSAD grant, USA), the Deutsche Multiple Sklerose Gesellschaft (DMSG) Bundesverband e.V. and Charité – Universitätsmedizin Berlin (Rahel-Hirsch scholarship).

References

1. Adebayo, J., Gilmer, J., Muelly, M., Goodfellow, I., Hardt, M., Kim, B.: Sanity checks for saliency maps. In: Bengio, S., Wallach, H., Larochelle, H., Grauman, K., Cesa-Bianchi, N., Garnett, R. (eds.) Advances in Neural Information Processing Systems 31, pp. 9505–9515. Curran Associates, Inc. (2018), http://papers.nips.cc/paper/8160-sanity-checks-for-saliency-maps.pdf
2. Alvarez-Melis, D., Jaakkola, T.S.: On the robustness of interpretability methods. arXiv preprint arXiv:1806.08049 (2018)
3. Bach, S., Binder, A., Montavon, G., Klauschen, F., Müller, K.R., Samek, W.: On pixel-wise explanations for non-linear classifier decisions by layer-wise relevance propagation. PLoS ONE **10**(7), 1–46 (2015). https://doi.org/10.1371/journal.pone.0130140
4. Bakker, R., Tiesinga, P., Kötter, R.: The scalable brain atlas: instant web-based access to public brain atlases and related content. Neuroinformatics **13**(3), 353–366 (2015)
5. Böhle, M., Eitel, F., Weygandt, M., Ritter, K.: Layer-wise relevance propagation for explaining deep neural network decisions in MRI-based Alzheimer's disease classification. Front. Aging Neurosci. **11**, 194 (2019). https://doi.org/10.3389/fnagi.2019.00194. https://www.frontiersin.org/article/10.3389/fnagi.2019.00194
6. Eitel, F., et al.: Uncovering convolutional neural network decisions for diagnosing multiple sclerosis on conventional MRI using layer-wise relevance propagation. CoRR (2019). http://arxiv.org/abs/1904.08771

7. Esmaeilzadeh, S., Belivanis, D.I., Pohl, K.M., Adeli, E.: End-to-end Alzheimer's disease diagnosis and biomarker identification. In: Shi, Y., Suk, H.-I., Liu, M. (eds.) MLMI 2018. LNCS, vol. 11046, pp. 337–345. Springer, Cham (2018). https://doi.org/10.1007/978-3-030-00919-9_39

8. Korolev, S., Safiullin, A., Belyaev, M., Dodonova, Y.: Residual and plain convolutional neural networks for 3D brain MRI classification. In: 2017 IEEE 14th International Symposium on Biomedical Imaging (ISBI 2017), pp. 835–838, April 2017. https://doi.org/10.1109/ISBI.2017.7950647

9. Liu, M., Cheng, D., Wang, K., Wang, Y.: The Alzheimer's disease neuroimaging initiative: multi-modality cascaded convolutional neural networks for Alzheimer's disease diagnosis. Neuroinformatics 16(3), 295–308 (2018). https://doi.org/10.1007/s12021-018-9370-4

10. Montavon, G., Lapuschkin, S., Binder, A., Samek, W., Müller, K.R.: Explaining nonlinear classification decisions with deep taylor decomposition. Pattern Recognit. 65, 211–222 (2017). https://doi.org/10.1016/j.patcog.2016.11.008. http://www.sciencedirect.com/science/article/pii/S0031320316303582

11. Montavon, G., Samek, W., Müller, K.R.: Methods for interpreting and understanding deep neural networks. Digit. Signal Process. 73, 1–15 (2018). https://doi.org/10.1016/j.dsp.2017.10.011. http://www.sciencedirect.com/science/article/pii/S1051200417302385

12. Rieke, J., Eitel, F., Weygandt, M., Haynes, J.-D., Ritter, K.: Visualizing convolutional networks for MRI-based diagnosis of Alzheimer's disease. In: Stoyanov, D., et al. (eds.) MLCN/DLF/IMIMIC -2018. LNCS, vol. 11038, pp. 24–31. Springer, Cham (2018). https://doi.org/10.1007/978-3-030-02628-8_3

13. Shrikumar, A., Greenside, P., Kundaje, A.: Learning important features through propagating activation differences. In: Proceedings of the 34th International Conference on Machine Learning-Volume 70, pp. 3145–3153. JMLR.org (2017)

14. Simonyan, K., Vedaldi, A., Zisserman, A.: Deep inside convolutional networks: visualising image classification models and saliency maps. arXiv preprint arXiv:1312.6034 (2013)

15. Springenberg, J., Dosovitskiy, A., Brox, T., Riedmiller, M.: Striving for simplicity: the all convolutional net. In: ICLR (Workshop Track) (2015). http://lmb.informatik.uni-freiburg.de/Publications/2015/DB15a

16. Sundararajan, M., Taly, A., Yan, Q.: Axiomatic attribution for deep networks. In: Proceedings of the 34th International Conference on Machine Learning - Volume 70, ICML 2017, pp. 3319–3328. JMLR.org (2017). http://dl.acm.org/citation.cfm?id=3305890.3306024

17. Vieira, S., Pinaya, W.H., Mechelli, A.: Using deep learning to investigate the neuroimaging correlates of psychiatric and neurological disorders: methods and applications. Neurosci. Biobehav. Rev. 74, 58–75 (2017). https://doi.org/10.1016/J.NEUBIOREV.2017.01.002. https://www.sciencedirect.com/science/article/pii/S0149763416305176

18. Zeiler, M.D., Fergus, R.: Visualizing and understanding convolutional networks. In: Fleet, D., Pajdla, T., Schiele, B., Tuytelaars, T. (eds.) ECCV 2014. LNCS, vol. 8689, pp. 818–833. Springer, Cham (2014). https://doi.org/10.1007/978-3-319-10590-1_53

UBS: A Dimension-Agnostic Metric for Concept Vector Interpretability Applied to Radiomics

Hugo Yeche[1,2,3]($\boxtimes$), Justin Harrison[1,4]($\boxtimes$), and Tess Berthier[1]($\boxtimes$)

[1] Imagia, Montreal, Canada
hg.yeche@gmail.com, justin.harrison@queensu.ca,
tess.berthier@imagia.com
[2] Eurecom, Sophia-Antipolis, France
[3] ENS Paris-Saclay, Paris, France
[4] Queen's University, Kingston, Canada

Abstract. Understanding predictions in Deep Learning (DL) models is crucial for domain experts without any DL expertise in order to justify resultant decision-making process. As of today, medical models are often based on hand-crafted features such as radiomics, though their link with neural network features remains unclear. To address the lack of interpretability, approaches based on human-understandable concepts such as TCAV have been introduced. These methods have shown promising results, though they are unsuited for continuous value concepts and their introduced metrics do not adapt well to high-dimensional spaces. To bridge the gap with radiomics-based models, we implement a regression concept vector showing the impact of radiomic features on the predictions of deep networks. In addition, we introduce a new metric with improved scaling to high-dimensional spaces, allowing comparison across multiple layers.

Keywords: Radiomics · Concept vector · Dimensionality · Interpretability

1 Introduction

The recent advances in Deep Learning (DL) have been rapidly changing the landscape in many domains, improving results significantly as new models are discovered. However, understanding the predictions of such models remains a challenge: their size and complexity make them difficult to interpret. This is especially true in healthcare applications, where explainability is essential for decision-making processes.

Recently, Radiomic [1] analysis has emerged as a methodology to obtain key predictive or prognostic information for cancer research. It consists of extracting hand-crafted features from a segmented region of interest (ROI) for precision diagnostic and treatment. Although Convolutional Neural Networks (CNNs)

© Springer Nature Switzerland AG 2019
K. Suzuki et al. (Eds.): ML-CDS 2019/IMIMIC 2019, LNCS 11797, pp. 12–20, 2019.
https://doi.org/10.1007/978-3-030-33850-3_2

have shown classification scores comparable to medical experts, their reliance on interpretable clinical concepts or handcrafted features remains unclear.

Interpretability in DL is mainly based on attribution techniques such as saliency maps [2,3]. They highlight the region of an image that influence the classifier's decision the most. However, such methods show limitations due to their pixel-wise approach [5,6].

To avoid pixel-level methods, [4] propose a human interpretable approach called Concept Activation Vector (CAV): a concept dataset is made by the user to extract a vector (CAV), which is then used to compute the importance of the concept for the network's decision. However, having a dataset of concepts is fairly uncommon and creating one introduces human-bias during the image-selection step.

This problem was addressed by [7] with RCV, a method replacing the classifier of CAV by a linear regression model when dealing with continuous metric concepts such as radiomics. [7] introduced the Br score, a more discriminating metric than the TCAV baseline [4]. However, this score is limited as its magnitude is dependent on the current layer as well as the other concepts. Furthermore, the Br score does not disentangle how well a concept is embedded in the layer's feature space from how important this concept is to the network's final prediction.

In this work, we introduce a new, layer-agnostic metric named the Uniform Unit Ball Surface Sampling metric (UBS) allowing to compare the magnitude of scores across all layers in a CNN, resulting in a clearer understanding of the effect of consistency on a concept's importance. In addition, we disentangle a concept's representation in a feature space from its impact on a network's prediction. From this we validate the importance of specific textural radiomic features in the classification of nodules for mammographic images.

2   Related Work and Notations

In the following section, we clarify the notation adopted in the paper while describing CAV [4] and RCV [7] approaches. For a layer l, f_l is the function mapping any input to l's feature space. For categorical concepts we build a set of images for each concept c, labelled X_c, and then we perform a classification task between $f_l(X_c)$ and $f_l(X_r)$, where X_r is a set of random images. For a continuous concept $c(.)$, we fit a linear regression between $f_l(X_{test})$ and $c(X_{test})$. For both categorical and continuous concepts, a concept vector $\mathbf{v}_l^c$ is then extracted. This is the normal vector to the classifier's hyperplane for categorical concepts and the direction-vector of the regression for the continuous one. Finally, to measure the impact of a concept c on predicting an image x with a label t, a sensitivity score $\mathbf{s}_{t,l}^C(x)$ is computed:

$$\mathbf{s}_{t,l}^C(x) = \nabla p_{t,l}(f_l(x)) \cdot v_l^C \qquad (1)$$

where $p_{t,l}$ is the function returning the model's prediction for a class t from the activations at a layer l. From this sensitivity score per image, both methods propose a different metric per concept, each with their own limitations. [4] introduce a TCAV baseline score such that:

$$TCAV_{bl}(C, l, t) = \frac{\sum_{x \in X_{test}} \delta_{\mathbf{s}_{t,l}^C(x) > 0}}{|X_{test}|} \tag{2}$$

where δ_H is equal to 1 if H is true and is 0 otherwise. Because of TCAV baseline's lack of discrimination, [7] introduce the Br score metric in the RCV approach:

$$Br(C, l, t) = R^2 \frac{\hat{\mu}}{\hat{\sigma}} \tag{3}$$

where R^2 comes from the regression fitting step and $\hat{\mu}$ and $\hat{\sigma}$ are the respective mean and variance from the $\mathbf{s}_{t,l}^C(X_test)$ distribution. A normalization per layer is then applied such that the highest magnitude is equal to 1, leading to dependencies between the magnitude scores of the concepts.

3   Methods

The RCV approach entangles how well a concept is embedded to its impact on the network's prediction: By multiplying the R^2 score with a function of the sensitivity score, it is no longer possible to retrace the incidence of each on the Br score. Thus, in our approach, we separate the way we build the concept vectors, measured by the R^2 metric, from the measurement of their impact on the class' prediction score, evaluated by our metric UBS.

3.1   Radiomics Extraction and Concept Vector Building

To extract radiomic features, [8] developed a python library, `pyradiomics`, used to compute them for grayscale images from a segmented region of interest (ROI). In this paper, we used the aforementioned library to extract all the 2D radiomic features.

The RCV approach is suited for continuous values, hence its application to radiomics. Every regression is fitted on a 10-fold splitting and evaluated by R^2 scoring on the test section of the data. For clarity purposes, we only consider radiomics with an average R^2 score above 0.6, and a UBS is computed for each. To compare the radiomic features, we compute the Br for all of them, however, we replace the sensitivity score with a cosine similarity as we focus on the direction of the derivative rather than its magnitude.

As it will be further explained in the "Dataset and Implementation Details" section, extracting shape-based radiomics in our dataset resulted in a R^2 score below 0.6. Consequently, we rejected them and focused on textural radiomics: Gray Level Cooccurrence Matrix (GLCM [12]).

3.2 UBS Metric

As previously mentioned, the Br score from [7] is concept-dependant whereas the TCAV baseline metric introduced in [4] isn't sufficiently discriminating. Both issues arise from the effects of dimensionality on the cosine similarity: its magnitude tends to zero as the dimension increases while its symmetry remains unchanged. To cope with this issue, the TCAV baseline score takes into account only the cosine's sign while the Br score normalizes each cosine similarity score by the highest magnitude score at a layer of interest, providing only a local solution.

To allow the comparison of concepts across all layers, a normalization of the cosine similarity that scales with the dimension of the space is required. A threshold for the cosine similarity score's magnitude is necessary to asses its relative significance while considering the current space's dimension. In Theorem 1, we propose an upper bound on the cosine's magnitude between a unit vector with a random direction and a fixed unit vector, which represents a concept vector. We then use this bound to normalize the cosine similarity magnitude to obtain a dimension-agnostic metric.

Theorem 1. *For* $\mathbf{u} \in \mathbb{R}^n$ *such that* $||\mathbf{u}||_2 = 1$ *and* $\mathbf{v}$ *a random vector from* $\{\frac{-1}{\sqrt{n}}, \frac{1}{\sqrt{n}}\}^n$ *we have:*

$$\mathbf{P}(|\cos(\mathbf{u}, \mathbf{v})| < \sqrt{\frac{\log(n)}{n}}) > 1 - \frac{1}{n}$$

Proof. For $\mathbf{u} \in \mathbb{R}^n$ and $\mathbf{v}$, a random vector from $\{\frac{-1}{\sqrt{n}}, \frac{1}{\sqrt{n}}\}^n$ sampled uniformly, let's consider a random variable $X = cos(\mathbf{u}, \mathbf{v})$, using that all the $\mathbf{v}_i$ are independent and centered as well as $||\mathbf{u}||_2 = ||\mathbf{v}||_2 = 1$:

$$\mathbf{E}(X) = \mathbf{E}(\sum_{i=1}^{n} \mathbf{u}_i \mathbf{v}_i) = \sum_{i=1}^{n} \mathbf{u}_i \mathbf{E}(\mathbf{v}_i) = 0 \tag{4}$$

$$\begin{cases} i = j \Rightarrow \mathbf{E}(\mathbf{v}_i \mathbf{v}_j) = \mathbf{E}(\frac{1}{n}) = \frac{1}{n} \\ i \neq j \Rightarrow \mathbf{E}(\mathbf{v}_i \mathbf{v}_j) = \mathbf{E}(\mathbf{v}_i)\mathbf{E}(\mathbf{v}_j) = 0 \end{cases} \tag{5}$$

$$\mathbf{V}(X) = \mathbf{E}(X^2) - \mathbf{E}(X)^2 = \mathbf{E}(X^2) = \sum_{i,j=1}^{n} \mathbf{u}_i \mathbf{u}_j \mathbf{E}(\mathbf{v}_i \mathbf{v}_j) = \sum_{i=1}^{n} \frac{\mathbf{u}_i^2}{n} = \frac{1}{n} \tag{6}$$

Once we have obtained values for $\mathbf{E}(X)$ and $\mathbf{V}(X)$ we apply the Chernoff bound to X such that:

$$\mathbf{P}(|X| < t) > 1 - e^{\frac{-t^2}{V(X)}} \tag{7}$$

for $t = \sqrt{\frac{\log(n)}{n}}$, we obtain the following bound:

$$\mathbf{P}(|\cos(\mathbf{u}, \mathbf{v})| < \sqrt{\frac{\log(n)}{n}}) > 1 - \frac{1}{n}$$

As a result, we have a bound with a probability $1 - \frac{1}{n}$ for the cosine similarity of a fixed vector with any vector from uniform distribution over $\{\frac{-1}{\sqrt{n}}, \frac{1}{\sqrt{n}}\}^n$, which is a good approximation for sampling uniformly from the unit ball surface in high dimension. As the dimension increases linearly, there is an exponential increase in the number of points from which the samples are taken as they are drawn from 2^n points.

With this normalization constant for the cosine similarity scores, we build our metric called the Uniform Unit Ball Surface Sampling metric (UBS):

$$\begin{cases} \mathbf{UBS}(C, l, t) = \frac{sign(C,l,t)}{|S_t|} \sum_{x \in S_t} \frac{|\cos(\nabla p_{t,l}(f_l(x)), v_l^C)|}{\sqrt{\frac{\log(n)}{n}}} \\ \mathbf{s.t}\ sign(C_t^l) = \frac{\sum_{x \in S_t} \cos(\nabla p_{t,l}(f_l(x)), v_l^C)}{|\sum_{x \in S_t} \cos(\nabla p_{t,l}(f_l(x)), v_l^C)|} \end{cases} \tag{8}$$

where n is the dimension at the layer l and S_t is the set of test images. Note that the sign is used due to the bound being based on the magnitude of the cosine. When using the UBS metric, only concepts with score magnitudes above 1 are considered relevant to the decision-making.

4   Experiments and Results

4.1   Dataset and Implementation Details

For our experiments, we used the publicly available dataset CBIS-DDSM (Curated Breast Imaging Subset of DDSM) [9,10]; a database of 1644 scanned film mammography study cases. The dataset contains calcifications and masses with their corresponding ROI segmentation.

500×500 px centered patches were made from the segmentation masks, the size is chosen through analysis of the variations in masses and calcifications size. Manual analysis of the generated patches was done to reject ineligible samples and improve accuracy. Rejected patches contained either masses that occupied the entire image, calcifications that were invisible when the image was re-sized to 224×224 px, or both calcifications and masses. When using the same test/train split as the original dataset, 155 calcifications + 179 masses were obtained for the test set and 743 calcifications + 557 masses were obtained for the train set.

Patches were re-sized to 224×224 px, normalized, and subjected to data augmentation (flipping and rotations) during the training phase. The used networks included a CNN of 3 convolution layers followed by 3 dense layers (CNN-3) and a Squeezenet v1.1 [11]. The networks were chosen not only for their high accuracy and speed, but also for their low number of layers, facilitating the concept per layer comparison (Figs. 1 and 3).

As shown in Fig. 2, the segmentations of the smaller calcifications are imprecise, encompassing groups of calcifications rather than individuals and generating a large margin around the area. The resulting segmentation is larger and more circular, making differentiating between single masses and clusters of calcifications based only on shape difficult. This makes it impossible to leverage the shape radiomics, a feature frequently used by experts for sample discrimination.

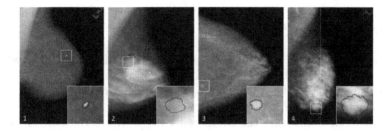

Fig. 1. Representative mammographic images from CBIS-DDSM. 1 and 2 being calcifications and 2 and 3 masses.

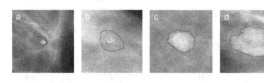

Model	Accuracy	AUC
CNN-3	0.87	0.95
Squeeze Net	0.93	0.98

Fig. 2. Representative patches, (a, b) being calcification and (c, d) being masses.

Fig. 3. Training Results for CNN-3 and SqueezeNet.

4.2 Concept Vector for Radiomic Features Results

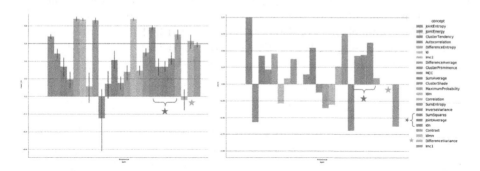

Fig. 4. Results at layer fire6/concat of SqueezeNet for GLCM radiomics, with corresponding R^2 scores (left) and Br scores (right) for calcification prediction. (Color figure online)

We first demonstrate that by not distinguishing between the R^2 score and the sensitivity score, we are unable to tell which factor has an impact on the magnitude of the Br score. Figure 4 illustrates the computed R^2 and Br scores on the fire6 layer of a SqueezeNet1.1 for the GLCM features on mammographic images. Two observations can be made from these results:

– The deviations between some Br scores can only be determined by the R^2 score variations, as seen with the three concepts denoted by the purple star.

– Contrastingly, some Br scores can only be determined by the sensitivity score, as shown with the *DifferenceVariance* (yellow star).

As the concepts are all normalized in-between themselves, it is impossible to assess their individual relevance. Two high-scoring concepts in two different layers will have the same maximum score, however this does not imply that they have the same impact on the final prediction.

Figures 5 and 6 illustrate the computed UBS scores of the GLCM features across several layers in a SqueezeNet v1.1 and CNN-3 for the same dataset. As previously mentioned, concepts with an R^2 score below 0.6 at the fitting step were rejected. As seen in Fig. 6, the plots for masses and calcifications are symmetric due to the binary nature of the classification task and the symmetry of the UBS metric. To emphasize the variation of scores across several layers in the SqueezeNet, we chose to only show the calcification results.

In Fig. 5, we demonstrate that our metric is not biased by the inner layer normalization. If bias was present, concepts such as DifferenceEntropy, DifferenceAverage and Contrast would have had a very high magnitude in the first layers, then would have dropped considerably on the last layer due to the importance of the JointEntropy, despite them being even more relevant.

With our UBS metric, we see that radiomic features describing increased entropy, such as DifferenceEntropy and JointEntropy, as well as those describing variations of intensity, such as Contrast and DifferenceAverage, shift the model's prediction towards calcifications. Conversely, radiomic features based on homogeneity such as *Id*, *Idm* and *InverseVariance* lead to an increased prediction of masses. These findings are consistent with those of [13,14]. The scores are also consistent across numerous layers regardless of dimension.

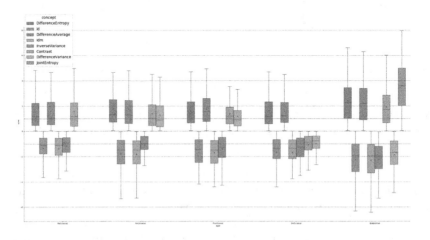

Fig. 5. UBS scores for layer fire2/concat to fire6/concat on SqueezeNet model for calcifications prediction. UBS scores are represented by the green points as the mean of each distributions (Color figure online)

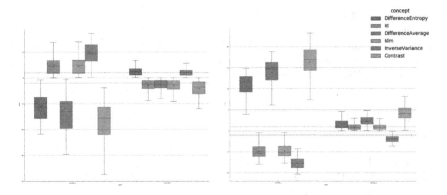

Fig. 6. UBS scores on the CNN-3, for calcifications (left) and masses (right) predictions. (Color figure online)

Finally, with the UBS metric it is observed that the last two convolutional layers of the CNN-3 contain large variations in the most important concepts in comparison with the SqueezeNet, which shows greater consistency across layers. This can be seen in Fig. 6 and is a possible explanation for the different classification scores between the two models.

5   Conclusion

In conclusion, the UBS metric shows a layer-agnostic behavior, allowing us to compare across all layers in the CNN. Not only it adds clarity to the concept's importance in the layers themselves, but it disentangles its representation in a feature space from its relevance in the network's prediction. Furthermore, applying UBS over mammographic images validated [13,14] the importance of specific textural concepts during the classification task, improving explainability as their impact is comparable across all the layers.

Overall, in this paper we proposed a proof of concept of the UBS metric over mammographic images, further works would involve applying our methodology to other datasets and different radiomic features, including examining shape-based radiomics we were unable to evaluate. In addition, the bound we uncovered in Theorem 1 can be improved to be more compatible with the smaller dimensions that are found in the final dense layers.

References

1. Lambin, P., et al.: Radiomics: extracting more information from medical images using advanced feature analysis. Eur. J. Cancer **48**, 441–446 (2012)
2. Simonyan, K., Vedaldi, A., Zisserman, A.: Deep inside convolutional networks: visualising image classification models and saliency maps. arXiv preprint arXiv:1312.6034 (2013)

3. Springenberg, J.T., Dosovitskiy, A., Brox, T., Riedmiller, M.: Striving for simplicity: the all convolutional net. arXiv preprint arXiv:1412.6806 (2014)
4. Kim, B., Gilmer, J., Wattenberg, M., Viégas, F.: TCAV: relative concept importance testing with linear concept activation vectors (2018)
5. Adebayo, J., Gilmer, J., Muelly, M., Goodfellow, I., Hardt, M., Kim, B.: Sanity checks for saliency maps. In Advances in Neural Information Processing Systems (2018)
6. Kindermans, P.J., et al.: The (un) reliability of saliency methods. arXiv preprint arXiv:1711.00867 (2017)
7. Graziani, M., Andrearczyk, V., Müller, H.: Regression concept vectors for bidirectional explanations in histopathology. In: Stoyanov, D., et al. (eds.) MLCN/DLF/IMIMIC 2018. LNCS, vol. 11038, pp. 124–132. Springer, Cham (2018). https://doi.org/10.1007/978-3-030-02628-8_14
8. Van Griethuysen, J.J., et al.: Computational radiomics system to decode the radiographic phenotype. Cancer Res. **77**, e104–e107 (2017)
9. Lee, R.S., Gimenez, F., Hoogi, A., Miyake, K.K., Gorovoy, M., Rubin, D.L.: A curated mammography data set for use in computer-aided detection and diagnosis research. Sci. Data **4**, 170177 (2017)
10. Heath, M., Bowyer, K., Kopans, D., Moore, R., Kegelmeyer, W.P.: The digital database for screening mammography. In: Proceedings of the 5th International Workshop on Digital Mammography (2000)
11. Iandola, F.N., Han, S., Moskewicz, M.W., Ashraf, K., Dally, W.J., Keutzer, K.: SqueezeNet: AlexNet-level accuracy with 50x fewer parameters and <0.5 MB model size. arXiv preprint arXiv:1602.07360 (2016)
12. Haralick, R.M., Shanmugam, K.: Textural features for image classification. IEEE Trans. Syst. Man Cybern. **6**, 610–621 (1973)
13. Huang, S.Y., et al.: Exploration of PET and MRI radiomic features for decoding breast cancer phenotypes and prognosis. NPJ Breast Cancer **4**, 24 (2018)
14. Parekh, V.S., Jacobs, M.A.: Integrated radiomic framework for breast cancer and tumor biology using advanced machine learning and multiparametric MRI. NPJ Breast Cancer **3**, 43 (2017)

Generation of Multimodal Justification Using Visual Word Constraint Model for Explainable Computer-Aided Diagnosis

Hyebin Lee[1], Seong Tae Kim[2], and Yong Man Ro[1](✉)

[1] Image and Video Systems Lab, School of Electrical Engineering,
KAIST, Daejeon, South Korea
{machipoe,ymro}@kaist.ac.kr
[2] Computer Aided Medical Procedures, Technical University of Munich,
Munich, Germany
seongtae.kim@tum.de

Abstract. The ambiguity of the decision-making process has been pointed out as the main obstacle to practically applying the deep learning-based method in spite of its outstanding performance. Interpretability can guarantee the confidence of the deep learning system, therefore it is particularly important in the medical field. In this study, a novel deep network is proposed to explain the diagnostic decision with visual pointing map and diagnostic sentence justifying result simultaneously. To increase the accuracy of sentence generation, a visual word constraint model is devised in training justification generator. To verify the proposed method, comparative experiments were conducted on the problem of the diagnosis of breast masses. Experimental results demonstrated that the proposed deep network can explain diagnosis more accurately with various textual justifications.

Keywords: Explainable deep learning · Textual justification · Visual explanation · Multimodal deep learning

1 Introduction

Thanks to the remarkable achievements of deep learning technology, Computer-aided detection (CADe) and Computer-aided diagnosis (CADx) show notable successes with deep learning based approaches [9,12]. On the contrary, difficulty in understanding the cause of a decision still remain as a dominant limitation for the application of deep learning based method in the real world. To cope with this problem, the multimodal approach [4] has been devoted to developing the

This work was supported by Institute for Information & communications Technology Planning & Evaluation(IITP) grant funded by the Korea government(MSIT) (No. 2017-0-01779, A machine learning and statistical inference framework for explainable artificial intelligence).

© Springer Nature Switzerland AG 2019
K. Suzuki et al. (Eds.): ML-CDS 2019/IMIMIC 2019, LNCS 11797, pp. 21–29, 2019.
https://doi.org/10.1007/978-3-030-33850-3_3

method for interpreting the decision via generating explanation in the form of attentive pointing map and text.

In medical applications such as CADx, the method with interpretability reflecting the reliability of result is more important, because it is mainly used in a high-risk environment directly connected to human health. There are several works which utilize additional information attached to the medical image for the decision explanation. [5,6] introduced a critic network which exploits pre-defined medical lexicon to elaborate visual evidence of the diagnosis. [22,24] proposed the networks generating natural medical reports from various Recurrent Neural Networks (RNNs) structure and pointing an informative area of input medical image.

However, it is challenging to generate accurate sentences with large variation because of the high complexity in the natural language. As addressed in [13], the conventional captioning methods suffer a problem in which the model duplicates a completely identical sentence of the training set even if the model is trained on the large dataset. Since the duplicated sentences only describe the portraits of training images, it cannot fully cover the variation of unseen images. This problem becomes more serious in the medical research area due to the limited number of medical report data.

In this study, we propose a novel deep network to provide visual and textual justification interpreting the diagnostic decision. The main contribution of this study is summarized as followings:

(1) We propose a new justification generator to interpret the diagnostic decision of the deep network. The proposed justification generator provides the textual and visual justification for the diagnostic decision. It can apply to any conventional CADx network (classifier of malignant mass and benign mass) to interpret the decision of the deep network without diagnostic performance degradation.

(2) To overcome the duplication problem in which the model generates a completely identical sentence of the training set, we devise a new learning method utilizing a visual word constraint loss. For evaluating the proposed method, a sentence dataset describing the characteristics (the shape and the margin) of breast masses has been collected in this study. Experimental results have shown that the proposed method can generate various textual justifications which have higher similarity with human-made sentences.

2   Proposed Method

2.1   Overall Framework

An overall proposed network framework is shown in Fig. 1. As shown in the figure, the overall architecture of the deep network was divided into two parts, a diagnosis network (any conventional CADx network) and a justification generator. The justification generator employed a visual feature and a diagnostic decision of the diagnosis network. To avoid the sentence duplication of the training set, a visual word constraint loss was devised in the training stage. The detailed structure of the justification generator and the learning strategy are described in the following subsections.

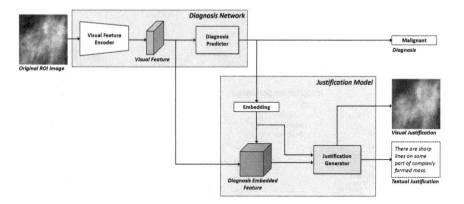

Fig. 1. Overall proposed deep network framework for producing textual justification and visual justification.

2.2 Justification Generator

As shown in Fig. 2, in order to explain the diagnostic decision, the justification generator made a textual justification and a visual justification from the diagnostic decision and the visual feature. From given image $\mathbf{I}(n, m)$, the visual feature $\mathbf{f}_v(n, m, k)$ was extracted by the visual feature encoder. Using $\mathbf{f}_v$ as input, the diagnosis predictor made a diagnostic decision $\hat{\mathbf{y}}_d = \{p_{benign}, p_{malignant}\}$. p_{benign} and $p_{malignant}$ denote the probability of the benign and the probability of the malignant, respectively. Afterward, $\hat{\mathbf{y}}_d$ was embedded to k-dim vector $\alpha_d^{embed}(k)$. It was weight of the channel attention refining visual feature:

$$\mathbf{f}_{embed}(n, m, k) = \mathbf{f}_v(n, m, k) \cdot \alpha_d^{embed}(k), \tag{1}$$

where $\mathbf{f}_{embed}$ denotes a diagnosis embedded feature and $\alpha_d^{embed}(k)$ is the k-th element of α_d^{embed}. Through multiple convolutional layers, multi-channel feature $\mathbf{f}_{embed}$ was encoded into single-channel 2D map $\alpha_{va}(n, m)$. The visual justification α_d^{vis} was generated as followings:

$$\alpha_d^{vis}(n, m) = \frac{\exp(\alpha_{va}(n, m))}{\sum_n \sum_m \exp(\alpha_{va}(n, m))}, \tag{2}$$

The softmax operation in Eq. (2) was conducted to represent more focused areas and suppress the activation on the background. For obtaining the textual justification, a text generating feature $\mathbf{f}_{text}$ was encoded from $\mathbf{f}_{embed}$. $\mathbf{f}_{text}$ was used as the input of the textual justification generator which was designed with the Long Short Term Memory (LSTM) module. The text generating feature $\mathbf{f}_{text}$ was obtained by

$$\mathbf{f}_{embed+vis}(n, m, k) = \mathbf{f}_{embed}(n, m, k) \cdot \alpha_d{}^{vis}(n, m) \cdot \alpha_d{}^{embed}(k), \qquad (3)$$

$$\mathbf{f}_{text} = \mathrm{T}_{\varphi_{test}}(\mathbf{f}_{embed+vis} + \mathbf{f}_{embed}), \qquad (4)$$

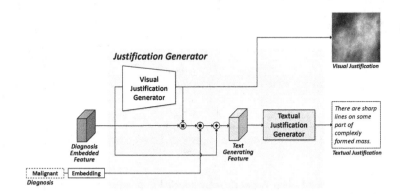

Fig. 2. Detailed architecture of the justification generator.

where $\mathbf{f}_{embed+vis}$ denotes the refined diagnosis embedded feature by the spatial attention with $\alpha_d{}^{vis}$ and the channel-wise attention with $\alpha_d{}^{embed}$. $\mathrm{T}_{\varphi_{test}}(\cdot)$ is a function with learnable parameter φ_{test} for encoding the text generating feature. $\mathrm{T}_{\varphi_{test}}(\cdot)$ was implemented by multiple convolutional layers. Finally, the textual justification $\mathbf{W} = [w_1, w_2, \cdots]$ was generated by using the two-hidden-layer-stacked LSTM network $f^{LSTM}(\cdot)$ as

$$h_t = f^{LSTM}(\mathbf{f}_{text}, w_{t-1}, h_{t-1}), \qquad (5)$$

where w_t denotes a t-th word obtained by converting the t-th hidden state h_t using a linear function with learnable parameters.

2.3   Network Training Using Visual Word Constraint

In the training stage, the textual difference loss $\mathcal{L}_D$ was calculated from cross-entropy loss function representing difference between the generated textual justification $\mathbf{W}$ and the ground truth of textual justification $\mathbf{W}^{GT}$. In order to overcome the aforementioned duplication problem in the textual justification generation, we devised a visual word constraint model $V_{con}(\cdot)$. A sentence classifier [7] was utilized to construct the visual word constraint model. Through the visual word constraint model, the margin and the shape were predicted from the given sentences $\mathbf{W}$ as

$$\hat{\mathbf{y}}_{con} = \{\hat{\mathbf{y}}_{ma}, \hat{\mathbf{y}}_{sh}\} = V_{con}(\mathbf{W}), \qquad (6)$$

where $\hat{\mathbf{y}}_{ma}, \hat{\mathbf{y}}_{sh}$ are a predicted margin and a predicted shape, respectively. The visual word constraint model was pre-trained on sentences of the training set and utilized to guide the textual justification generator with a visual word constraint loss $\mathcal{L}_C$ as

$$\mathcal{L}_C = \text{cross-entropy}(\hat{\mathbf{y}}_{ma}, \mathbf{y}_{ma}^{GT}) + \text{cross-entropy}(\hat{\mathbf{y}}_{sh}, \mathbf{y}_{sh}^{GT}), \tag{7}$$

where $\mathbf{y}_{ma}^{GT}, \mathbf{y}_{sh}^{GT}$ are ground truth of margin and shape. As a result, overall network was trained by minimizing following loss function:

$$\mathcal{L} = \mathcal{L}_D + \alpha \mathcal{L}_C, \tag{8}$$

where α is a balancing hyper-parameter. By introducing visual word constraint loss, the textual justification can contain more various words. The proposed model can also grasp similarity in meaning with the word describing the same margin or shape even without an additional large word set embedding to vector space.

3 Experiments

3.1 Experimental Condition

In the experiments, we used two mammogram datasets. The first dataset was the public mammogram dataset, named Digital Database for Screening Mammography (DDSM) dataset [3]. The BI-RADS descriptions and the location of masses were annotated by the radiologist [3]. The dataset (605 masses) was split into a training set (484 masses) and a test set (121 masses). The second dataset was the Full-Field Digital Mammogram (FFDM) dataset from a hospital. A total of 147 masses of 67 patients were collected and two-fold cross-validation was conducted in this study. The deep network learned from the DDSM dataset was used as the initial network for training with the FFDM dataset.

The sentence datasets were collected on both the DDSM dataset and the FFDM dataset. Since BI-RADS mass lexicons (margin and shape) are widely used to describing breast mass by medical doctors and closely related to malignancy of the mass, we comprised sentences based on these lexicons. To make sentence various and be close to the description of medical doctors, we investigated words and phrases, which describe margin and shape in the medical papers and books [1,10,14,16,17,19,20], and its synonyms called visual words. Visual words of each lexicon included 4–12 words or phrases. Three sentences were annotated for each ROI mass image and each sentence contained at least one visual word for mass margin and shape respectively. According to [4], every sentence included at least 10 words and did not contain BI-RADS mass lexicon as it is. In addition, the sentences contained individual details.

In order to increase the number of training data, data augmentation was conducted. The two sizes of patches were cropped from the original ROI image at five locations (top left, top right, center, bottom left, bottom right).

Each cropped image was also flipped and rotated (0°, 90°, 180°, and 270°). The size of mini-batch was set to 64 and an Adam optimizer [8] was used with learning rate 0.0005. The balancing parameter was empirically set to 2.

For the diagnosis network at the front part of the proposed network, we used VGG16 [18] based binary classifier. The weights of the pre-trained network with ImageNet [2] was utilized as initial weights and the fine-tuning was conducted. As the visual feature $\mathbf{f}_v(n, m, k)$, the feature map after conv 5_3 in the VGG16 network was used in this study. The area under the ROC curve (AUC) was calculated for evaluating the diagnostic performance and the AUC of 0.918 was obtained from the trained diagnosis network on the DDSM dataset. During the training of the justification generator, the parameters of the diagnosis network were fixed.

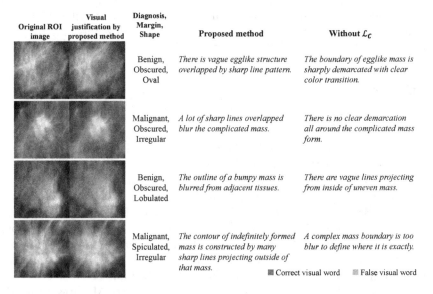

Fig. 3. Results of the textual and the visual justification of the proposed method. Diagnosis, margin, and shape denote ground truth. The sentences for textual justification are compared with the proposed method and the method learned without $\mathcal{L}_C$.

3.2   Results

To validate the effect of our model, we compared the proposed method with the method learned without visual word constraint loss $\mathcal{L}_C$. Figure 3 shows the examples of the generated visual justification and the textual justification. As shown in the figure, the proposed method can provide the textual justification and the visual justification for the diagnostic decision. The sentences generated by the method learned without visual word constraint loss $\mathcal{L}_C$ were also compared. $\mathcal{L}_C$ enabled the textual justification generator to match the margin and shape labels of the generated texture justification and input ROI mass image in the training phase. Therefore, the generated textual justification was more accurate in the proposed method compared to the method without $\mathcal{L}_C$.

For quantitatively evaluating the quality of the textual justification, we adopted BLEU [15], ROUGE-L [11], and CIDEr [21] metrics which calculated the similarity between the generated sentence and the reference (ground truth) sentence. Table 1 shows the results of the evaluation for the textual justification on the DDSM and the FFDM datasets in terms of BLEU, ROUGE-L, and CIDEr. As shown in the table, with the proposed method of learning the model utilizing $\mathcal{L}_C$, the generated textual justifications were closer to reference sentences composed by a human. Furthermore, following the evaluations in [23], the ratio of the unique sentences and the ratio of the novel sentences were calculated in Table 2 on the DDSM and the FFDM datasets. The unique sentence was defined as the sentence which was not repeated in all generated sentences and the novel sentence was defined as the sentence which was unseen in the training set. These two metrics were calculated to evaluate the textual justification regarding the duplication problem. If duplication occurred, the textual justification could not accurately narrate the given test image. By calculating the ratio of the novel and unique sentences, it was possible to measure how reliably the textual justification was generated according to the given image. As shown in the table, the number of novel sentences was dramatically improved with the proposed method. The number of the unique sentences in the proposed method was also increased compared to the method learned without $\mathcal{L}_C$.

Table 1. Evaluation of textual justification on the DDSM and FFDM dataset.

	DDSM dataset		FFDM dataset	
	Proposed method	Without $\mathcal{L}_C$	Proposed method	Without $\mathcal{L}_C$
BLEU-1	**0.3870**	0.3687	**0.4070**	0.3835
BLEU-2	**0.1968**	0.1742	**0.2296**	0.2133
BLEU-3	**0.1026**	0.0887	**0.1354**	0.1187
BLEU-4	**0.0586**	0.0490	**0.0871**	0.0650
ROUGE_L	**0.2526**	0.2439	**0.2650**	0.2596
CIDEr	**0.1514**	0.1469	**0.1366**	0.1185

Table 2. Ratios of the unique sentences and the novel sentences on the DDSM and FFDM dataset.

	DDSM dataset		FFDM dataset	
	Proposed method	Without $\mathcal{L}_C$	Proposed method	Without $\mathcal{L}_C$
Ratio of unique sentence	**93.39%**	64.46%	**54.42%**	11.56%
Ratio of novel sentence	**43.80%**	4.13%	**65.99%**	8.16%

4   Conclusion

In this paper, we proposed the novel deep network to provide multimodal justification for the diagnostic decision. The proposed method can explain the reason for the diagnostic decision with the sentence and indicate the important areas on the image. In the case of textual justification generation for medical purposes, the network tended to generate templated results due to the limited number of medical reports. To overcome this problem, the learning method utilizing visual word constraint loss was devised. By the comparative experiments, the effectiveness of the proposed method was verified. The proposed method generated more diverse and accurate textual justifications. These results imply that the proposed method can explain the diagnostic decision of the deep network more persuasively. As future work, it would be a meaningful direction to evaluate the effectiveness of the multimodal explanation in terms of helping users better trust and understand CADx outputs.

References

1. Berment, H., Becette, V., Mohallem, M., Ferreira, F., Chérel, P.: Masses in mammography: what are the underlying anatomopathological lesions? Diagn. Intervent. Imag. **95**(2), 124–133 (2014)
2. Deng, J., Dong, W., Socher, R., Li, L., Li, K., Fei-Fei, L.: Imagenet: a large-scale hierarchical image database. In: CVPR, pp. 248–255. IEEE (2009)
3. Heath, M., Bowyer, K., Kopans, D., Moore, R., Kegelmeyer, W.: The digital database for screening mammography. In: International Workshop on Digital Mammography, pp. 212–218. Medical Physics Publishing (2000)
4. Huk Park, D., et al.: Multimodal explanations: justifying decisions and pointing to the evidence. In: CVPR, pp. 8779–8788. IEEE (2018)
5. Kim, S., Lee, J., Lee, H., Ro, Y.: Visually interpretable deep network for diagnosis of breast masses on mammograms. Phys. Med. & Biol. **63**(23), 235025 (2018)
6. Kim, S., Lee, J., Ro, Y.: Visual evidence for interpreting diagnostic decision of deep neural network in computer-aided diagnosis. In: Medical Imaging 2019: Computer-Aided Diagnosis, vol. 10950, p. 109500K. International Society for Optics and Photonics (2019)
7. Kim, Y.: Convolutional neural networks for sentence classification. In: Conference on Empirical Methods in Natural Language Processing, pp. 1746–1751 (2014)
8. Kingma, D., Ba, J.: Adam: a method for stochastic optimization. ICLR (2015)
9. Kooi, T., Litjens, G., Van Ginneken, B., Gubern-Mérida, A., Sánchez, C.I., Mann, R., den Heeten, A., Karssemeijer, N.: Large scale deep learning for computer aided detection of mammographic lesions. Med. Image Anal. **35**, 303–312 (2017)
10. Lee, K., Talati, N., Oudsema, R., Steinberger, S., Margolies, L.: Bi-rads 3: current and future use of probably benign. Current Radiol. Rep. **6**(2), 5 (2018)
11. Lin, C.: Rouge: a package for automatic evaluation of summaries. Text Summarization Branches Out (2004)
12. Litjens, G., Kooi, T., Bejnordi, B.E., Setio, A.A.A., Ciompi, F., Ghafoorian, M., Van Der Laak, J.A., Van Ginneken, B., Sánchez, C.I.: A survey on deep learning in medical image analysis. Med. Image Anal. **42**, 60–88 (2017)

13. Liu, X., Li, H., Shao, J., Chen, D., Wang, X.: Show, tell and discriminate: image captioning by self-retrieval with partially labeled data. In: ECCV (2018)
14. Moon, W., Lo, C., Chang, J., Huang, C., Chen, J., Chang, R.: Quantitative ultrasound analysis for classification of bi-rads category 3 breast masses. J. Digital Imag. **26**(6), 1091–1098 (2013)
15. Papineni, K., Roukos, S., Ward, T., Zhu, W.: Bleu: a method for automatic evaluation of machine translation. In: Annual Meeting of the Association for Computational Linguistics. pp. 311–318 (2002)
16. of Radiology, A.C.: Breast Imaging Reporting and Data System® (BI-RADS®). American College of Radiology, Reston, Va, 4 edn. (2003)
17. Selvi, R.: Breast Diseases Imaging and Clinical Management. Springer India, New Delhi (2015)
18. Simonyan, K., Zisserman, A.: Very deep convolutional networks for large-scale image recognition. In: ICLR (2015)
19. Surendiran, B., Vadivel, A.: Mammogram mass classification using various geometric shape and margin features for early detection of breast cancer. Int. J. Med. Eng. Inform. **4**(1), 36–54 (2012)
20. Thomassin-Naggara, I., Tardivon, A., Chopier, J.: Standardized diagnosis and reporting of breast cancer. Diagn. Interv. Imag. **95**(7–8), 759–766 (2014)
21. Vedantam, R., Lawrence Zitnick, C., Parikh, D.: Cider: Consensus-based image description evaluation. In: CVPR, pp. 4566–4575. IEEE (2015)
22. Wang, X., Peng, Y., Lu, L., Lu, Z., Summers, R.: Tienet: text-image embedding network for common thorax disease classification and reporting in chest x-rays. In: CVPR, pp. 9049–9058. IEEE (2018)
23. Wang, Y., Lin, Z., Shen, X., Cohen, S., Cottrell, G.: Skeleton key: image captioning by skeleton-attribute decomposition. In: CVPR, IEEE (2017)
24. Zhang, Z., Xie, Y., Xing, F., McGough, M., Yang, L.: Mdnet: a semantically and visually interpretable medical image diagnosis network. In: CVPR, pp. 6428–6436. IEEE (2017)

Incorporating Task-Specific Structural Knowledge into CNNs for Brain Midline Shift Detection

Maxim Pisov[1,2], Mikhail Goncharov[2,3], Nadezhda Kurochkina[1],
Sergey Morozov[4], Victor Gombolevskiy[4], Valeria Chernina[4],
Anton Vladzymyrskyy[4], Ksenia Zamyatina[4], Anna Chesnokova[4], Igor Pronin[5],
Michael Shifrin[5], and Mikhail Belyaev[1,2(✉)]

[1] Skolkovo Institute of Science and Technology, Moscow, Russia
`m.belyaev@skoltech.ru`
[2] Kharkevich Institute for Information Transmission Problems, Moscow, Russia
[3] Moscow Institute of Physics and Technology, Moscow, Russia
[4] Center for Diagnostics and Telemedicine, Moscow, Russia
[5] Burdenko Neurosurgery Institute, Moscow, Russia

Abstract. Midline shift (MLS) is a well-established factor used for outcome prediction in traumatic brain injury, stroke and brain tumors. The
importance of automatic estimation of MLS was recently highlighted
by ACR Data Science Institute. In this paper we introduce a novel deep
learning based approach for the problem of MLS detection, which exploits
task-specific structural knowledge. We evaluate our method on a large
dataset containing heterogeneous images with significant MLS and show
that its mean error approaches the inter-expert variability. Finally, we
show the robustness of our approach by validating it on an external
dataset, acquired during routine clinical practice.

Keywords: Neural networks · Midline shift · Interpretability ·
Confidence

1 Introduction

The brain midline can be viewed as a line on axial and coronal projections
of diverse imaging modalities (Fig. 1, left). As the human brain is approxi-
mately symmetrical, the midline is straight in healthy subjects. However, various
pathological conditions, such as traumatic brain injuries (TBI), stroke and brain
tumors, may break this symmetry and lead to midline shift (MLS) [8].

A major number of studies show that MLS has a prognostic value for outcome
prediction of various brain pathologies: level of consciousness in patients with
acute intracranial hematoma [16], median survival in patients with glioblastoma

---

The original version of this chapter was revised: the names of two authors and the
grant number were corrected. The correction to this chapter is available at https://doi.
org/10.1007/978-3-030-33850-3_11

ⓒ Springer Nature Switzerland AG 2019
K. Suzuki et al. (Eds.): ML-CDS 2019/IMIMIC 2019, LNCS 11797, pp. 30–38, 2019.
https://doi.org/10.1007/978-3-030-33850-3_4

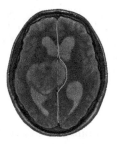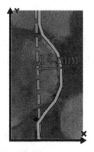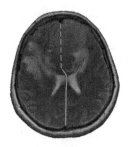

Fig. 1. Left: an axial slice from a MRI image with corresponding midline (red) and a hypothetical normal midline (blue, dashed). Center: the midline shift. Right: a dubious case with an ill-defined midline (red, dashed). (Color figure online)

multiforme [3], the outcome in patients with TBI [5]. Overall, early identification of patients with severe midline shift would assist patients management [14].

However, definitions of significant MLS vary across studies. While the 5 millimeters (mm) threshold is frequently used, other approaches are common. For example, MLS larger than 9 mm was identified in [14]; the 5 mm threshold was not justified within [5]. Such diversity is partly explained by the absence of a robust objective methodology of MLS estimation. A recent study [13] suggests that interrater variability of MLS estimation is rather high (intraclass correlation coefficients 0.72–0.89).

The importance of MLS estimation and the need for its automation was recently highlighted by The American College of Radiology Data Science Institute [10], and some promising results have already been achieved in this area (Sect. 3). In this paper we propose a novel deep learning based approach[1] for the MLS detection task. We show that combining a standard segmentation approach with task-specific structural knowledge yields results which are more accurate, compared to straightforward CNNs for regression, and also interpretable, since the key part of the method is the midline localization. Moreover, we show that our method generalizes well on highly heterogeneous data and provide a natural way of estimating its confidence.

2   Problem

We define the midline on an axial slice as a vertical curve that separates the brain hemispheres (Fig. 1, left). The midline shift for an axial slice is then defined as the maximal distance between the midline (which might be deformed) and a hypothetical normal midline (Fig. 1, center). Finally, the midline shift for a whole brain is the maximal midline shift across all axial slices where the midline is present. **The task** is to determine, for a given brain image, the midline shift as well as the corresponding axial slice on which it is manifested.

---

[1] Full code for training and inference is available at GitHub: https://github.com/neuro-ml/midline-shift-detection.

It is worth noting that in some complicated cases even professional radiologists cannot confidently determine the localization of the midline (Fig. 1, right). Taking into account such dubious cases, it is also desirable that the method for MLS detection has a means of estimating its own confidence.

3   Related Work

Most of the methods for automatic MLS estimation are computer vision (CV) based and rely on keypoints detection. The proposed approaches often have a lot of "moving parts" which makes them hard to implement and fine-tune. For example, in [9] the authors use a four-step pipeline (edge detection, morphological filtering, lines detection, rule-based filtering) just to detect the cerebral falx. Another drawback of keypoints-based methods is that they require various important regions to be present on the image, e.g. many methods can be applied only to slices that contain ventricles [1] which makes them inapplicable to cases where the midline shift is manifested on lower or higher slices.

There are also a few papers that propose deep learning methods. In [2] the authors trained an adapted a version of ResNet to classify whether there is a significant midline shift on a given slice. Another interesting approach that combines deep learning with classical CV is described in [6]. Here the authors use a U-Net [15] architecture for brain extraction, cisterns and acute intracranial lesions segmentation, while MLS detection is based on keypoints.

4   Method

A straightforward deep learning approach is to directly predict the MLS via a convolutional neural network. Following the authors of [2], we tested a ResNet-based [4] network which predicted the MLS for each axial slice of given image. The final prediction was obtained as the maximal MLS only among the slices that contained an annotated midline. However, even in such a simplified design (the model did not need to filter out the slices for which the MLS was undefined), this method yields poor results as we show in Sect. 7.

Our intuition behind this is that the midline shift is a very high-level concept: the network needs to learn to detect several keypoints located very far from each other (Fig. 1), as well as take into account their relative positions. The latter is a particularly difficult task for convolutional neural networks due to their invariance to translation.

On the contrary, the midline has visual features, like continuity and local symmetry, that are distinguishable on a smaller scale. This brings us to the idea to reduce the task of MLS prediction to the task of midline estimation: for a given slice we localize the midline while exploiting the structural knowledge about the target, then we derive the MLS from the predicted curve based on the definition given in Sect. 2. Normal midline is estimated as a straight line between prediction endpoints.

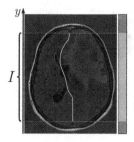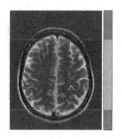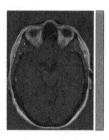

Fig. 2. The binary masks of the regions where the midline is defined (red). Note the rightmost image, for which the midline is undefined everywhere. (Color figure online)

The key structural facts are: (1) for each coordinate y there is at most one x-coordinate, which is refered as **midline**$_y$, such that the pixel (**midline**$_y, y$) is situated on the midline; (2) **midline**$_y$ exists only for y-coordinates within certain interval I on the Oy axis to which binary mask we refer as **limits** (Fig. 2).

These facts imply that our method must be capable of solving the regression problem of **mildine** estimation and the classification problem of **limits** prediction. To solve these tasks, we propose a two-headed convolutional neural network with shared input layers (Fig. 3). As loss function, we optimize a weighted combination of standard losses for regression and classification:

$$ L = \lambda_1 \cdot \frac{1}{|I|} \sum_{y \in I} (\textbf{midline}_y - \textbf{midline}_y^{\text{pred}})^2 + \lambda_2 \cdot \text{BCE}(\textbf{limits}, \textbf{limits}^{\text{pred}}), $$

where **midline**$_y^{\text{pred}}$ and **limits**^{pred} are the network's predictions, BCE is binary cross-entropy.

4.1 Midline Estimation

In order to estimate the midline we adapt a segmentation approach. In a standard setting (with sigmoid activation and binary cross entropy loss) the output can be interpreted as "independent" probability of a particular pixel to be situated on the midline. In this case the **midline** is obtained after applying argmax along the Ox axis.

However, as we show in Sect. 7, significantly better results can be achieved while imposing the following constraint on the output probability map

$$ \sum_x \textbf{output}_{xy}^{\text{midline}} = 1, \tag{1} $$

which follows from the structural fact (1). Next, taking into account that for any given y-coordinate the head's output represents a probability distribution, we propose to predict the midline as its expected value:

$$ \textbf{midline}_y^{\text{pred}} = \sum_x x \cdot \textbf{output}_{xy}^{\text{midline}}. $$

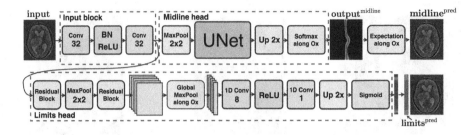

Fig. 3. Schematic representation of the proposed architecture.

The overall architecture for midline estimation is shown in Fig. 3 (top). For our experiments we chose a UNet-based [15] architecture as a de facto standard for medical image segmentation. We replaced plain convolutional layers by residual blocks [4] which are considered to improve the performance, as suggested by [11]. Also, during feature maps concatenation we use linear interpolation to make the output's shape equal to the input's shape. Finally, we apply a softmax nonlinearity to the network's output along the Ox axis (instead of sigmoid), which ensures that the constraint from (1) is respected. Note that because the head's output represents a probability distribution, at inference time we can calculate various statistics based on this distribution, e.g. percentiles, which are needed to estimate confidence intervals. This is a very important aspect of our approach which gives us a natural means of estimating the model's uncertainty.

4.2 Limits Prediction

Since the proposed midline estimation approach yields $\mathbf{midline}_y^{\mathrm{pred}}$ for all y-coordinates, we need to filter out the predicted values for the regions where the midline is not defined (Fig. 2, hatched). The corresponding limits are obtained by thresholding the second head's output ($\mathbf{limits}^{\mathrm{pred}}$) and taking the convex hull.

The architecture of the second head is shown in Fig. 3 (bottom). It has the same input layers as the midline estimation network, which are followed by two residual blocks [4]. Next, a global max pooling is applied along the Ox axis in order to reduce the dimensionality of the 2D feature maps to 1D. Finally we apply two 1D convolutions followed by the sigmoid activation function.

5   Experimental Setup

At train time in all of our experiments we used Adam optimizer [7] with default parameters ($\beta_1 = 0.9, \beta_2 = 0.999$) and a learning rate of 10^{-3}, which showed the best results on the validation set. We used equal ($\lambda_1 = \lambda_2 = 1$) weights in the final loss as we didn't notice any loss imbalance at train time.

Also, we applied a simple preprocessing in order to reduce the data variability: resampling the axial slices to a 0.5×0.5 mm pixel spacing, background removal by Otsu thresholding [12] and intensity normalization to zero mean and unit variance. Additionally, at train time we used random flips along the Ox axis as a cheap data augmentation technique.

The training was performed on batches of size 40 (which was simply determined by the amount of available GPU memory), until the validation scores reached a plateau, which happened at approx. 32000 batches. For this reason we used 32000 iterations for all our experiments.

6   Data

In our experiments we used data from two sources.

The first dataset (DS1) consists of 352 MRI series that come from a neurosurgery hospital and belong to patients with severe brain damage caused by tumors: 64% of the images have a significant midline shift (≥ 5 mm), the mean MLS is 7.8 ± 5.0 mm. The dataset was labeled by an experienced neuroradiologist (exp1) and three specialists with limited background in neuroradiology (exp2-4). Their inter- and intra-expert variability is shown in Table 2. We split this dataset using 5-fold cross-validation. For each fold, we additionally leave 8 images out the training set to form a validation set.

The second dataset (DS2) comes from an out-patient clinic and represents a homogeneous sample of 203 MRI series acquired in routine clinical practice. For this dataset only the MLS is available but not the midline itself; only 8% of images have a large MLS (≥ 5 mm), the mean MLS is 2.9 ± 1.5 mm. We use this dataset only for final models' quality assessment in a prospective fashion.

The series from both sources contain only axial slices but have various voxel spacings, ranging from $0.2 \times 0.2 \times 1$ mm to $1 \times 1 \times 5$ mm, and modalities: T1 (25%), T2 (68%) and FLAIR (7%). The images were collected using scanners from GE/Siemens and Toshiba/Siemens for DS1 and DS2 respectively.

7   Results

7.1   Midline Shift Detection

We compare the proposed method with a direct MLS regression via ResNet [4] on two tasks: (1) MLS prediction; (2) significant MLS (≥ 5 mm) detection. In order to evaluate the quality of both methods we use mean absolute error (MAE) and the area under the ROC-curve (ROC AUC) for task 1 and 2 respectively. The ROC-curve was obtained by thresholding the predicted MLS by different values (from 0 to maximal MLS magnitude). The results are presented in Table 1.

Table 1. Midline shift detection scores for various models (± std) calculated on 5-fold cross-validation.

	MAE, mm		ROC AUC	
	DS1	DS2	DS1	DS2
ResNet-152	2.92 ± 3.15	1.84 ± 1.10	0.91 ± 0.03	0.80 ± 0.04
Proposed	**1.54 ± 1.98**	**0.75 ± 0.04**	**0.95 ± 0.02**	**0.92 ± 0.02**

7.2 Midline Estimation

In order to assess the midline estimation performance we use root-mean-square error (RMSE) as well as maximal error (MAX):

$$\mathrm{RMSE}(\mathbf{midline}_y, \mathbf{midline}_y^{\mathrm{pred}}) = \sqrt{|I|^{-1} \sum_{y \in I} (\mathbf{midline}_y - \mathbf{midline}_y^{\mathrm{pred}})^2},$$

$$\mathrm{MAX}(\mathbf{midline}_y, \mathbf{midline}_y^{\mathrm{pred}}) = \max_{y \in I} |\mathbf{midline}_y - \mathbf{midline}_y^{\mathrm{pred}}|.$$

These metrics, averaged along axial slices (MAXs, RMSEs) as well as entire brain images (MAX, RMSE), are shown in Table 2.

Table 2. Top: midline estimation metrics (± std) calculated on 5-fold cross-validation for DS1. Bottom: neuroradiologist (exp1) variability on DS1.

	MAX	RMSE	MAXs	RMSEs
Segmentation	7.45 ± 9.84	0.95 ± 0.61	2.12 ± 3.25	0.81 ± 0.64
Proposed	3.61 ± 2.62	0.79 ± 0.44	1.58 ± 1.39	0.69 ± 0.54
exp1 vs exp1	3.16 ± 2.16	0.66 ± 0.19	1.47 ± 1.05	0.62 ± 0.50
exp1 vs exp2-4	3.44 ± 2.13	0.77 ± 0.35	1.47 ± 0.97	0.66 ± 0.19

We compare our method with a naïve segmentation approach mentioned in Sect. 4.1. Note that plain segmentation performs significantly worse in terms of maximal error, which is a more important characteristic for MLS detection.

8   Discussion

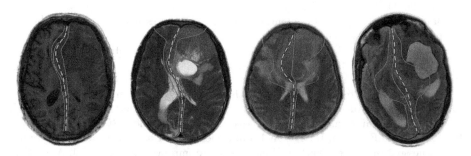

Fig. 4. Ground-truth (red) and predicted (yellow, dashed) midlines with their 95% confidence intervals for 2 random samples (left) and 2 typical examples from the set of cases with the largest errors (right). (Color figure online)

Figure 4 (right) shows several examples on which our method performs poorly. Our analysis of such examples suggests that the main source of errors are some really complicated cases that even professional radiologists have doubts with, e.g. images on which the tumor is located directly in the middle of the brain, or incorrect cases with an extracerebral tumor located in the medial longitudinal fissure, e.g. falx meningioma. Note how in the areas of greatest error the model's uncertainty is much higher.

Our preliminary experiments with CT images show that the proposed method can be easily adapted to work with CT, however we require a larger dataset to support this claim, which might be the subject of our future work.

Acknowledgements. The development of the interpretable algorithm (done by M. Pisov and M. Goncharov) was supported by the Russian Science Foundation grant 17-11-01390.

References

1. Chen, W., Belle, A., Cockrell, C., Ward, K.R., Najarian, K.: Automated midline shift and intracranial pressure estimation based on brain CT images. J. Visualized Exp. JoVE **74**, e3871 (2013)
2. Chilamkurthy, S., et al.: Deep learning algorithms for detection of critical findings in head ct scans: a retrospective study. Lancet **392**(10162), 2388–2396 (2018)
3. Gamburg, E.S., Regine, W.F., Patchell, R.A., Strottmann, J.M., Mohiuddin, M., Young, A.B.: The prognostic significance of midline shift at presentation on survival in patients with glioblastoma multiforme. Int. J. Radiat. Oncol.* Biol.* Phys. **48**(5), 1359–1362 (2000)
4. He, K., Zhang, X., Ren, S., Sun, J.: Deep residual learning for image recognition. In: Proceedings of the IEEE Conference on Computer Vision and Pattern Recognition, pp. 770–778 (2016)

5. Jacobs, B., Beems, T., van der Vliet, T.M., Diaz-Arrastia, R.R., Borm, G.F., Vos, P.E.: Computed tomography and outcome in moderate and severe traumatic brain injury: hematoma volume and midline shift revisited. J. Neurotrauma **28**(2), 203–215 (2011)

6. Jain, S., et al.: Automatic quantification of CT features inacute traumatic brain injury. J. Neurotrauma (2019)

7. Kingma, D.P., Ba, J.: Adam: a method for stochastic optimization. arXiv preprint arXiv:1412.6980 (2014)

8. Liao, C.C., Chen, Y.F., Xiao, F.: Brain midline shift measurement and its automation: a review of techniques and algorithms. Int. J. Biomed. Imaging (2018)

9. Liu, R., et al.: Automatic detection and quantification of brain midline shift using anatomical marker model. Comput. Med. Imaging Graphics **38**(1), 1–14 (2014)

10. McGinty, G.B., Allen, B.: The ACR data science institute and AI advisory group: harnessing the power of artificial intelligence to improve patient care. J. Am. College Radiol. **15**(3), 577–579 (2018)

11. Milletari, F., Navab, N., Ahmadi, S.A.: V-net: fully convolutional neural networks for volumetric medical image segmentation. In: 2016 Fourth International Conference on 3D Vision (3DV), pp. 565–571. IEEE (2016)

12. Otsu, N.: A threshold selection method from gray-level histograms. IEEE Trans. Syst. Man Cybern. **9**(1), 62–66 (1979)

13. Paletta, N., Maali, L., Zahran, A., Sethuraman, S., Figueroa, R., Nichols, F.T., Bruno, A.: A simplified quantitative method to measure brain shifts in patients with middle cerebral artery stroke. J. Neuroimaging **28**(1), 61–63 (2018)

14. Pullicino, P.M., Alexandrov, A., Shelton, J., Alexandrova, N., Smurawska, L., Norris, J.: Mass effect and death from severe acute stroke. Neurology **49**(4), 1090–1095 (1997)

15. Ronneberger, O., Fischer, P., Brox, T.: U-net: convolutional networks for biomedical image segmentation. In: Navab, N., Hornegger, J., Wells, W.M., Frangi, A.F. (eds.) MICCAI 2015. LNCS, vol. 9351, pp. 234–241. Springer, Cham (2015). https://doi.org/10.1007/978-3-319-24574-4_28

16. Ross, D.A., Olsen, W.L., Ross, A.M., Andrews, B.T., Pitts, L.H.: Brain shift, level of consciousness, and restoration of consciousness in patients with acute intracranial hematoma. J. Neurosurg. **71**(4), 498–502 (1989)

Guideline-Based Additive Explanation for Computer-Aided Diagnosis of Lung Nodules

⋅Peifei Zhu[(✉)] and Masahiro Ogino

Research and Development Group, Hitachi, Ltd., Tokyo, Japan
peifei.zhu.ww@hitachi.com

Abstract. Machine Learning (ML) models have achieved remarkable predictive capability in Computer-Aided Diagnosis (CAD) systems. However, a problem of such models is that they are regarded as black-box models and lack of an explicit representation. In this work, a Guideline-based Additive eXplanation (GAX) framework is proposed for interpreting ML-based CAD systems. A medical guideline standardizes decision making in disease diagnosis. The idea of GAX is generating understandable explanations according to the criteria of the guideline. It contains two steps: anatomical features defined on the basis of the guideline are first generated using rule-based segmentation and anatomical regularities, and perturbation-based analysis is then used for calculating the importance of each feature. In addition, global explanation is also obtained by analyzing the entire dataset, where measurements are calculated from anatomical features, and a figure containing the overview of which measurements are important is generated. The proposed GAX is evaluated on a lung CT image dataset. The results demonstrate that GAX can provide understandable explanations to gain trust in clinical practice, and also present data bias for users to further improve the model.

1 Introduction

Machine learning (ML) have demonstrated tremendous success in various application domains. In medical domains, ML based Computer-Aided Diagnosis (CAD) systems have been developed to assist clinicians in detecting and classifying nodules. Such systems may be able to reduce inter-observer variability and improve decision making in image diagnosis. On the other hand, the growing availability of big data has increased the benefits of using complex models, which brings a trade-off between accuracy and interpretability. This becomes a serious problem in medical domains because it would be irresponsible to trust predictions of a black-box system by default. Every decision should be made accessible for appropriate validation by clinicians. Therefore, interpretability is absolutely necessary to build systems with high reliability.

Various methods have been recently proposed to address the black-box issue. These methods can be categorized into two types: (1) inherently interpretable

© Springer Nature Switzerland AG 2019
K. Suzuki et al. (Eds.): ML-CDS 2019/IMIMIC 2019, LNCS 11797, pp. 39–47, 2019.
https://doi.org/10.1007/978-3-030-33850-3_5

models [1,2] and (2) post-hoc analysis to provide additive insights. Since the type one method usually needs to modify the algorithm and retrain the model, users who already have a high performance model might prefer to use the type two method. Saliency method [3–5] which visualizes ML predictions by highlighting important pixels is a popular post-hoc method. A limitation of such method is the vulnerability to the changes of input image intensity. Activation Maximization [6,7] method synthesize images to maximally.invert a latent representation. This method has a problem that it visualizes a model overall so there is no prediction for specific input images. Perturbation-based method uses the perturbation of data points [8,9] or features [10,11] to check how the model's response changes. A limitation is the region of interest it picks up might not have a understandable meaning for the users.

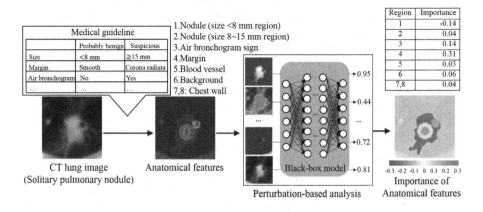

Fig. 1. Framework of GAX for lung nodule diagnosis.

This work proposed a Guideline-based Additive eXplanation (GAX) method to provide insights of a black-box model's prediction for CT lung nodule classification. A medical guideline is aimed for guiding decisions and criteria regarding diagnosis, management, and treatment. For lung cancer CT, the American College of Radiology presented a "Lung-RADS" guideline [12] to standardize nodule classification. The idea of GAX is generating understandable explanations according to the guideline. A framework of GAX is shown in Fig. 1.

In GAX, anatomical features such as size, margin, and air bronchogram, are first generated according to the criteria of the guideline. These features are generated automatically by a combination of rule-based segmentation and anatomical regularities. Second, kernel SHAP [11] based perturbation analysis is used for calculating the importance of each feature. As a result, an importance map showing the impact of each feature is generated. In addition, global explanation is also obtained by analyzing the entire dataset, where measurements are selected and calculated from anatomical features, and a figure containing the overview of which measurements are important is generated.

This work has two major contributions. First, it proposes GAX which incorporates guideline criteria to generate anatomical features (major difference from SHAP) and use perturbation analysis to generate the feature importance. This idea can be applied to any CAD system to provide understandable explanations. Second, it presents both local and global explanations, not only providing additive explanations to gain trust in clinical practice, but also giving sights to further improve the model.

2   Guideline-Based Additive eXplanation (GAX)

2.1   Anatomical Feature Generation

According to the "Lung-RADS" guideline [12], features such as size, margin, air bronchogram sign, are important to differentiate between benign and malignant nodules. A way to interpret and verify the black-box model is to check whether such anatomical features are important for a prediction or not. Therefore, our first target is to segment regions with anatomical meaning. To avoid the black-box problem happen in the segmentation, no learning method is used. Unlike nature images, medical images always have anatomical regularities, i.e. similar structures, components, and such regularizes are extremely important in improving segmentation performance. In this work, a two-step segmentation method is proposed, where an intensity-based method called Watershed [13] is first used to extract all possible regions, and the anatomical regularities are used to improve each region as well as standardize each region label.

Watershed segmentation contains two steps. First, each pixel is connected to its lowest neighbor pixel, and all pixels connected to same lowest neighbor pixel are made as a region. Second, the region merging method [14] which merges most similar pair of adjacent regions is used as the post-processing to remove noise. The results usually suffer from three problems: (1) nodule and chest wall cannot be segmented as seperated regions, (2) air bronchogram is regarded as noise, and (3) standardized label for each region is difficult to generalize. The anatomical regularities are used to solve these problems.

For problem 1, since the connections between nodule and chest wall are usually narrow shapes, morphological opening operator with a radius kernel can be used to remove the connections. To preserve the nodule margin, the following process is also applied. The region before and after the opening operation is define as A and B. Once the nodule and chest wall region are separated, the space C between these two can be regarded as background. Finally, OR operation is applied between A and B (C is excluded) to recover the nodule margin.

Problem 2 can be solve by applying the noise reduction (second step of Watershed) outside the nodule. Please note most of the nodules is centered at the image patch because the detection is usually designed to extract the bounding-box of the nodules. Therefore, the nodule region can be easily located by searching the largest region around the center, and air bronchogram can be determined by searching small regions with low intensity inside the nodule.

For the label standardization in problem 3, the nodule, chest wall and air bronchogram have already been determined. Size less than 8 mm and size 8–15 mm region of the nodule (if existed) can also be easily determined by image resolution and the center coordinate of the nodule. Small regions with high intensity outside the nodule is determined as the blood vessel, and the remained region is the background.

2.2 Perturbation-Based Analysis

Perturbation-based method uses perturbation to verify the change of the model's output. This work is based on Kernel SHAP [11] which uses sparse linear models as explanations. The details are as follows.

An explainable sparse linear model is defined as g, and the complexity of g is denoted as $\Omega(g)$. For linear models, $\Omega(g)$ means the number of non-zero weights. The original representation of an instance is x, and a binary vector indicating "presence" or "absence" is x'. A black-box model is defined as f. In classification, $f(x)$ is the probability that x belongs to a certain class. A proximity measure between an instance z and x is denoted as $\pi_x(z)$. A loss enforces the faithfulness of the explanation model g to the black-box model f is defined as $L(f, g, \pi_x)$. The explanation can be produced by the following:

$$\xi(x) = \mathrm{argmin} L(f, g, \pi_x) + \Omega(g) \tag{1}$$

In order to be model-agnostic, it is necessary to minimize the loss L without any assumption about f. One way to approximate the loss L is to randomly sample features, denoted as z', from the binary vector representation x', and recovered in the original space z. Then the perturbed sample z passes through the black-box model and generates probability $f(z)$. Given the perturbed sample and the associated probability, an explanation $\xi(x)$ can be optimized.

On the other hand, since g is a sparse linear model, $g(z') = w \cdot z'$ can be denoted, where w is the importance of each feature. The local kernel $\pi_x(z)$ can be determined by shapely value estimation. Let M be the number of the features, the loss can be represented as:

$$L(f, g, \pi_x) = \Sigma \pi_x(z)(f(z) - w * z')^2 \tag{2}$$

$$\pi_x(z) = \frac{(M - 1)}{(M\,choose\,|z'|)|z'|(M - |z'|)} \tag{3}$$

In this work, an improvement has been made in feature sampling. Since most models cannot handle arbitrary missing data during the sampling, the "missing" is simulated by replacing the feature with some values. To generate more realistic samples, instead of using constant values, the background region segmented in Sect. 2.1 is used to fill the missing value for each test.

2.3   Global Explanation Generation

The local explanation can provide sights of a specific input data, while the global explanation verifies and assesses the entire dataset. This work proposed a global explanation method, where measurements are calculated from anatomical features, and a figure containing the overview of which measurements are important for the model is generated. Examples are shown in Sect. 3.2.

Five measurements are selected: nodule roughness, nodule diameter and air bronchogram size which are strongly related to the classification, chest wall location and background area which almost have no relation with the classification. Nodule diameter, air bronchogram size and background area can be easily calculated from the segmentation result. Nodule roughness is standard deviation of the distances from the nodule center to the nodule contour. As for chest wall location, the perimeter of the image patch is first divided into 12 equal parts, and the image center and the division points are connected to divide the image into 12 parts (clock-wise). Next, the geometric center of the chest wall is calculated, and chest wall location is the location of the geometric center in $k \in (1, 12)$ part.

The process contains (1) calculating each feature importance, (2) calculating each measurement, (3) drawing pairs of importance and measurement in a figure, and (4) repeating for every test image. In the cases where features such as air bronchogram and chest wall do not exist, the measurement and the importance are set as 0. Although the measurement and feature are not matched one-to-one, i.e. nodule roughness and nodule diameter come from same feature, the figure still gives an overview of which feature has large impact on the prediction.

3   Experiments

The proposed method is evaluated on a lung CT image dataset (LIDC-IDRI) that is available in [15]. This database contains 1018 cases with nodule annotations. Since our target is to interpret the classification results of benign and malignant, nodule patches are extracted from lung images in advance. There are 2650 images patches with a size of 64 * 64 pixels and a resolution of 1 mm * 1 mm being extracted. These patches are annotated as benign or malignant by experts. Since some of the comparison methods can only be applied to deep learning models, a same VGG16 model is used for all methods. The experiments are run in a NVIDIA GeForce GTX 1080 GPU, and the running time of GAX is about 0.5 s per image.

3.1   Additive Explanations to Gain Trust

In this experiment, GAX is compared with three widely used interpret methods: LIME [10], SHAP [11] and Grad-CAM [4]. Both LIME and SHAP use superpixel method to segment features, and the number of feature is set as the same with GAX. For Grad-CAM, the gradient information of the last convolutional layer is used to generate a heat-map. Comparison results are shown in Fig. 2.

In this example, the input image is classified as malignant with a probability of 99.8%. For each result except Grad-CAM (only shows important areas), red areas increase the probability of malignant, and green areas decrease the probability. The result of LIME and SHAP suffer from a problem that the region of interest they pick up do not have an understandable meaning for the humans. The result of Grad-CAM has a tendency that high intensity areas are easily picked up as important areas. GAX is able to provide an understandable explanation, i.e. margin and air bronchogram have positive influence for malignant class.

The consistency of the generated explanation with human intuition is also compared. Reference features, i.e. margins shown in Fig. 3(a), is annotated according to the guideline. They are considered as important features for classifying nodules. On the other hand, the region of top 1 feature is extracted for LIME, SHAP and GAX, and the top 20% important region is extracted for Grad-CAM. For each prediction on the test set, the fraction of the reference features recovered by the explanations are calculated. The average recall over all test samples are shown in Fig. 3(b). Since the Grad-CAM approach is likely to focus on the high intensity region, it has the lowest recall. The results of LIME and SHAP are comparable, however, since the features extracted are lack of anatomical meanings, the overall recall is low. The proposed GAX provides 86.2% recall, demonstrating the consistency with human intuition.

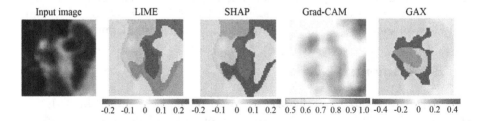

Fig. 2. An example of explanation result by 4 different methods.

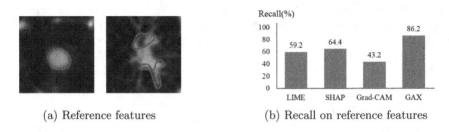

(a) Reference features   (b) Recall on reference features

Fig. 3. Consistency between explanations and reference features.

3.2   Insights to Improve the Model

In order to train a desirable model, data bias is usually one of the serious problems to overcome. However, this problem can be difficult to detect just by checking the raw data and predictions. In this experiment, a biased dataset is first generated, and GAX is then evaluated whether it can provide some insights to detect the bias. To generate a biased dataset, 100 images with chest wall on the right are picked up from malignant set, and 100 images with chest wall on the left are picked up from benign set. These image are used to train a VGG16 model. During the test, 100 images without bias are used, and two examples are shown in Fig. 4. In (a), the image is classified as malignant with a probability of almost 100%. Compare to Fig. 2, a difference is that the chest wall on the right shows a much larger influence. In (b), the image is also classified as malignant but with a probability of 58%. The chest wall on the left shows a large negative influence on malignant classification.

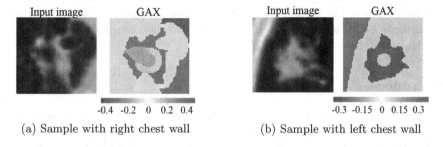

(a) Sample with right chest wall   (b) Sample with left chest wall

Fig. 4. Explanation results showing the influence of data bias.

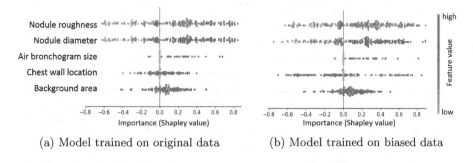

(a) Model trained on original data   (b) Model trained on biased data

Fig. 5. Example of global explanation result. (Color figure online)

Global explanations are generated by the method in Sect. 2.3. For comparison, the model trained on the original dataset and the biased dataset are both evaluated. The results for malignant classification are shown in Fig. 5. The color of point represents the measurement value (red high, blue low). For the original dataset in Fig. 5(a), high value of nodule roughness, diameter and air bronchogram size have positive influence on malignant classification, while chest wall and background have much less influence. For the biased dataset in Fig. 5(b), the influence of chest wall location becomes much larger, where high value (7 to 12 o'clock direction: chest wall on the left) shows negative influence and low value (1 to 6 o'clock direction: chest wall on the right) shows positive influence. The biased chest wall location is successfully detected, therefore, GAX might be useful for helping users to detect data bias and further improve the model.

4   Conclusions

In this work, a novel guideline-based explanation framework is proposed for interpreting black-box models in CAD systems. To the best of our knowledge, this is the first work that incorporating medical guidelines to generate understandable explanations for black-box model. As a major contribution, GAX can provide additive explanations to gain trust in clinical practice, and also present data bias to further improve the model. As a future direction, we plan to further evaluate the influence of features such as solid and ground-glass component that cannot be extracted in this work but are important.

References

1. Caruana, R., Lou, Y., Gehrke, J., Koch, P., Sturm, M., Elhadad, N.: Intelligible models for healthcare: predicting pneumonia risk and hospital 30-day readmission. In: the 21st ACM SIGKDD International Conference on Knowledge Discovery and Data Mining, pp. 1721–1730 (2015)
2. Letham, B., Rudin, C., McCormick, T.H., Madigan, D.: Interpretable classifiers using rules and bayesian analysis: building a better stroke prediction model. Ann. Appl. Stat. **9**(3), 1350–1371 (2015)
3. Simonyan, K., Vedaldi, A., Zisserman, A.: Deep inside convolutional networks: visualising image classification models and saliency maps. arXiv:1312.6034 [cs], December 2013. arXiv:1312.6034
4. Selvaraju, R.R., Cogswell, M., Das, A., Vedantam, R., Parikh, D., Batra, D.: Grad-CAM: visual explanations from deep networks via gradient-based localization. In: International Conference on Computer Vision (ICCV), pp. 618–626 (2017)
5. Dabkowski, P., Gal, Y.: Real time image saliency for black box classifiers. In: Advances in Neural Information Processing Systems (NIPS), pp. 6967–6976 (2017)
6. Mahendran, A., Vedaldi, A.: Understanding deep image representations by inverting them. In: International Conference on Computer Vision and Pattern Recognition (CVPR), pp. 5188–5196 (2015)
7. Mahendran, A., Vedaldi, A.: Visualizing deep convolutional neural networks using natural pre-images. Int. J. Comput. Vis. **120**(3), 233–255 (2016)
8. Koh, P.W., Liang, P.: Understanding black-box predictions via influence functions. In: International Conference on Machine Learning (ICML), pp. 1885–1894 (2017)
9. Zhang, C., Bengio, S., Hardt, M., Recht, B., Vinyals, O.: Understanding deep learning re-quires rethinking generalization. In: International Conference on Learning Representations (2017)

10. Ribeiro, M.T., Singh, S., Guestrin, C.: Why should I trust you? Explaining the predictions of any classifier. In: 22nd ACM SIGKDD International Conference on Knowledge Discovery and Data Mining, pp. 1135–1144 (2016)
11. Lundberg, S., Lee, S.: A unified approach to interpreting model predictions. In: Advances in Neural Information Processing Systems (NIPS), pp. 4765–4774 (2017)
12. American College of Radiology: Lung CT screening reporting and data system (Lung-RADS). American College of Radiology, Reston, VA (2014)
13. Nguyen, H.T., Worring, M., Van Den Boomgaard, R.: Watersnakes: energy-driven water-shed segmentation. IEEE Trans. Pattern Anal. Mach. Intell. **25**(3), 330–342 (2003)
14. Haris, K., Efstratiadis, S.N., Maglaveras, N., Katsaggelos, A.K.: Hybrid image segmentation using watersheds and fast region merging. IEEE Trans. Image Process. **7**(12), 1684–1699 (1998)
15. Armato III, S.G., et al.: The lung image database consortium (LIDC) and image database resource initiative (IDRI): a completed reference database of lung nodules on CT scans. Med. Phys. **38**(2), 915–931 (2011)

Deep Neural Network or Dermatologist?

Kyle Young[1], Gareth Booth[1], Becks Simpson[2], Reuben Dutton[1],
and Sally Shrapnel[1(✉)]

[1] School of Mathematics and Physics, University of Queensland, Brisbane, Australia
`s.shrapnel@uq.edu.au`
[2] Montreal Institute for Learning Algorithms, Montreal, Canada

Abstract. Deep learning techniques have proven high accuracy for identifying melanoma in digitised dermoscopic images. A strength is that these methods are not constrained by features that are pre-defined by human semantics. A down-side is that it is difficult to understand the rationale of the model predictions and to identify potential failure modes. This is a major barrier to adoption of deep learning in clinical practice. In this paper we ask if two existing local interpretability methods, Grad-CAM and Kernel SHAP, can shed light on convolutional neural networks trained in the context of melanoma detection. Our contributions are (i) we first explore the domain space via a reproducible, end-to-end learning framework that creates a suite of 30 models, all trained on a publicly available data set (HAM10000), (ii) we next explore the reliability of GradCAM and Kernel SHAP in this context via some basic sanity check experiments (iii) finally, we investigate a random selection of models from our suite using GradCAM and Kernel SHAP. We show that despite high accuracy, the models will occasionally assign importance to features that are not relevant to the diagnostic task. We also show that models of similar accuracy will produce different explanations as measured by these methods. This work represents first steps in bridging the gap between model accuracy and interpretability in the domain of skin cancer classification.

Keywords: Deep learning · Explainability · Melanoma

1 Introduction

Skin cancer is the most common form of cancer in the United States [11,17], and melanoma is the leading cause of skin cancer related death [18]. Automated diagnosis of melanoma from digitized dermoscopy images thus represents an important potential use case for deep learning methods. Inspired by a breakthrough result by Esteva et al., [7], many recent publications claim "better than dermatologist" performance of convolutional neural networks (CNNs) on a variety of skin cancer classification tasks [3,4,7–9,13]. If indeed such models have diagnostic performance comparable to board certified dermatologists, this heralds a new era in skin cancer care, with standardization of diagnosis and democratization

© Springer Nature Switzerland AG 2019
K. Suzuki et al. (Eds.): ML-CDS 2019/IMIMIC 2019, LNCS 11797, pp. 48–55, 2019.
https://doi.org/10.1007/978-3-030-33850-3_6

of access [10,14]. Early diagnosis of melanoma is associated with improved outcomes but poor availability of well trained clinicians in many parts of the world means too often diagnosis is made too late. CNNs represent an important new technology to address this problem for social good.

How can we evaluate the veracity of these exciting new claims? Unfortunately, privacy constraints typically make it difficult to access training, validation, test data, and final model weights. This makes it impossible to verify the accuracy of these published models and reproduce their claims [4]. As is common in medical settings, there are inherent *known* biases in the data: lesion classes are unevenly distributed, healthy images are over-represented, racial bias is present (few lesions are from dark-skinned individuals) [3] and there is significant variability in ground truth labelling [6]. Can we be confident the model has not inherited any of these known biases? A further challenge is due to the presence of *unknown* biases in the data. If an artifact is present in images from two diagnostic classes but more prevalent in one, how do we know when the model classifications are weighted by the presence or absence of this artifact?

In light of these problems, it is an open question as to the best strategy to determine if a given model will generalize to future data where the distribution of these biases may be different. Currently there are two approaches: (i) ad hoc techniques that penalize model complexity (batch normalization and dropout, for example), and (ii) training and testing models on larger and more complex data sets. Importantly, neither of these techniques can identify, nor correct, specific biases prior to model deployment.

In this paper, we investigate the possibility that current interpretability methods may assist in this task. Interpretability methods seek to produce an indication of features of the input data that the model regards as important for weighting the final diagnostic decision. While they do not capture the entirety of the predictive process, they can nonetheless provide some guidance to how a given model makes decisions.

2   Experiments

2.1   Data

For this study we use publicly available data from HAM10000, a well curated data set of dermoscopy images collected specifically for use in the machine learning context [22]. The full data set includes seven classes of skin lesions—in this study we concentrate on differentiating between benign naevus (moles) and melanoma, a particularly challenging clinical task. Our data set contains a total of 6017 images, with significant class imbalance: 5403 naevi and 614 malignant melanoma. We retain a balanced set of 200 images of each class as a hold out test set. It is worth noting that in the clinical context false negatives (predicting naevus when ground truth is melanoma) have far more serious consequences than false positives (predicting melanoma when ground truth is naevus). This means we need to ensure the class imbalance is addressed during training: a model trained and tested on the current distribution can achieve high accuracy (88%) simply by always guessing naevus.

2.2   Models

The majority of publications in this area use transfer learning from Inception, pre-trained on Imagenet with an added pooling layer, dense layer and dropout—we follow suit for ease of comparison. We address class imbalance by first augmenting the melanoma images, obtaining a final set of 1656 melanoma images. We then sample 15 random subsets of 818 images from both classes and train a total of 30 models via a Bayesian hyper-parameter search—searching over learning rate, dropout, momentum, $beta_1$, $beta_2$, number of dense nodes, number of epochs, SGD and Adam[1]. The aim is to survey the landscape of possible models, giving us a selection of multiple networks to compare and explore rather than a single, cherry-picked one. The mean AUC over the 30 models is 85% with a variance of 1.8% and a mean recall of 87%—a performance comparable to other published models in this context (e.g. the model of [9] achieved AUC of 86%)[2]. Reported AUC for melanoma identification from dermoscopy images for dermatologists is around 79% [9] and for primary care physicians even lower [16]. These results signal the fact that this is indeed a difficult task for which CNN decision support may prove useful.

It is interesting to note that the variance across model accuracy (AUC) over the 30 models is relatively small at 1.8%. While these models share the same basic architecture, they have been trained on different sub-samples of the data using different hyper-parameters—thus are likely converging on different local optima. This is evidenced by the differences in mis-classified test images across the different models. Interestingly, seventeen images were consistently mis-classified: at least 25/30 models got the class label wrong. For example, the naevus in Fig. 1 was mis-classified by all 30 models as melanoma. Interestingly, this lesion does arguably satisfy one of the clinical criteria for melanoma. A small human evaluation trial by 3 primary care physicians suggests these images are challenging: scores were 4/17, 5/17 and 6/17.

2.3   GradCAM and Kernel SHAP

GradCAM [19] and Kernel SHAP [12] are both model agnostic, local interpretability methods. While both highlight pixels that the trained network deems relevant for the final classification, they work in very different ways. GradCAM

---

[1] Details of augmentation, random data sampling, Bayesian hyper-parameter search, all code for training and experiments, including the final 30 trained models can be found here: https://github.com/KyleYoung1997/DNNorDermatologist.

[2] Note that differences in test set size and distribution mean that direct comparison of model performance via AUC is of limited merit. However, as AUC is the standard metric reported in the literature, we include it here. Further comment can be found in the conclusions.

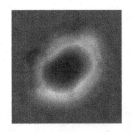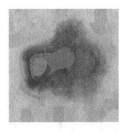

Fig. 1. Naevus mis-classified by all 30 models as a melanoma, with GradCAM and kernel SHAP saliency maps. Note there is more than one type of network within the lesion, a feature which can be a marker for melanoma. The GradCAM map (centre image) highlights a key deficiency of the method in this context: almost all of the lesion is obscured by the saliency map, rendering the "explanation" clinically meaningless.

computes the gradient of the class-score (logit) with respect to the feature map of the final convolutional layer. Formally, consider each input image as a vector $x \in R_d$ where our model is a function $S : R_d \rightarrow R_c$, with C the total number of classes. GradCAM provides an "interpretability" map $I : R_d \rightarrow R_d$ that maps inputs to objects of the same dimension. If A_k are feature maps obtained from the last convolutional layer, global average pooling of the gradients gives us a set of neuron importance maps $\alpha_c^k = \frac{1}{Z} \sum_i \sum_j \frac{\partial S}{\partial A_{ij}^k}$ and the final mask corresponds to a ReLU applied to a weighted linear combination of the feature maps and the importance maps: $I(x) = \text{ReLU}(\sum_k \alpha_c^k A^k)$. More details and examples can be found in [19].

While there are a large variety of methods for applying saliency maps, recent work has shown that many are in fact independent of both the model weights and/or the class labels [2]. In these cases it is likely the model architecture itself is constraining the saliency maps to look falsely meaningful: frequently the maps just act as a variant of edge detector [2]. This is particularly dangerous in the context of skin cancer detection as features at the borders of lesions are often considered diagnostic for melanoma: saliency maps that highlight the edges of a lesion may be misconstrued as clinically meaningful. We use GradCAM in our analysis because it was one of the few methods that passed the recommended sanity checks (we also perform our own to double-check this particular context).

We also investigate the use of Kernel SHAP [12], an interpretability method that was not among those investigated in [2], but has strong theoretical justification [15]. A stronger agreement was found between Shapley explanations and human explanations when compared to two alternative popular saliency methods, LIME and DeepLIFT [12], further confirming that this is an appropriate method to explore. Based on Shapley values from co-operative game theory [20], the method assigns a fair attribution value to each feature based on the contribution that feature makes to the total prediction. The method is proven to be the unique mapping that satisfies a number of reasonable criteria and is calculated by considering interactions between all possible subsets of features. For d features, calculating the Shapley value for a given feature k will need to account for all 2^{d-1} subsets containing k. Thus a downside to the original approach is that it scales exponentially in the number of features. Consequently, we use an approximate, computationally feasible method: Kernel SHAP [12].

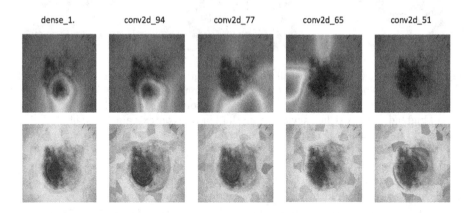

Fig. 2. Explanations following randomization of selected layers in the model. Changes demonstrate dependence of explanation on model weights. SSIM scores averaged over all images for GradCAM degraded across layers by 23%, 4%, 3%, 2%, 4%. Differences were also seen for kernel SHAP: 17%, 3%, 5%, 3%, 7%. Green signifies areas of positive contribution to a diagnosis of melanoma, red signifies negative. (Color figure online)

2.4 Sanity Checks

We perform three simple sanity checks on GradCAM and Kernel SHAP to explore their performance in this context. (i) **Reproducibility:** we run the algorithms twice using the same randomly selected model and the same image, then compare images visually and using SSIM[3]. GradCAM saliency maps were unsurprisingly visually identical, with a perfect SSIM of 1, reflecting the deterministic nature of this algorithm. Kernel SHAP images were visually close to identical, but with SSIM less than perfect (mean 0.92, standard deviation 0.028). This small deviance is unsurprising given the method requires approximation via random sampling of subsets of features. (ii) **Model dependence:** using techniques inspired by [2] we randomize the weights of selective, progressively shallower layers in a randomly chosen model and recompute the GradCAM and Kernel SHAP images. The idea is to ensure that the saliency maps are not in fact independent of model weights. Visual comparison and SSIM scores verify that the maps are indeed model dependent, an example can be seen in Fig. 2. (iii) **Sensitivity:** we compare saliency maps from three models with the same AUC. This test serves to determine the sensitivity of the maps to model weights and also provides insight into differences across models of similar performance. Visual inspection shows variation across three models with identical AUCs of 85% for

---

[3] Details on SSIM (Structural Similarity Index) can be found in [23].

both methods, with average variation in SSIM of 20% for both GradCAM and kernel SHAP. An example can be seen in Fig. 3.

2.5   Spurious Correlation

The saliency maps show that at this resolution the majority of images do not unambiguously capture clinically meaningful information. However, several images suggest that the model is indeed weighting the classification decision using spurious correlations. Notable examples include those images that highlight the dark corners of the images (e.g. Fig. 3).

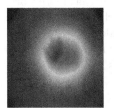 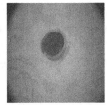  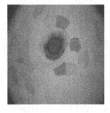

Fig. 3. GradCAM and kernel SHAP from two models with AUC 85%. Model 1 correctly predicted melanoma with 0.999 confidence (first two images). Model 2 incorrectly predicted naevus with 0.996 confidence (second two images). The saliency maps indicate model 2 has learned to weight the class decision using a spurious correlation: the dark corners of the image.

2.6   Limitations

There are a number of limitations of this study. The small data size makes overfitting more likely, thus increasing the chances that we would uncover spurious correlations. Additionally, while our small data size made many tasks computationally and practically feasible, for large test data sets this will not be the case—visual inspection to screen for spurious correlations will likely become impractical. An alternative approach would be to use these methods to provide feedback at the time of prediction: while a saliency map located on the lesion can not yet be viewed as justification that clinically meaningful correlations have been learned, a map that is clearly located on a clinically irrelevant region could be used to signal a prediction that should be ignored. Our study was also limited to models of a particular architecture, while we justify this as providing a point of comparison with existing published research, future work could include model architecture as a search hyper-parameter.

While the accuracy of our models is good and comparable to human accuracy, it is likely ensembled methods will improve accuracy further. It is difficult to envision how these interpretability methods could be applied meaningfully in this context. One alternative could be to use the maps themselves to regularize each of the models during training—methods such as GradMask suggest this may be possible [21]. Finally, there exists recent, alternative methods for implementing Shapley analysis that may well produce better results and permit the use of higher resolution images [1,5]. These experiments we leave for the future.

3 Conclusions

There is a significant literature comparing the performance of DNNs and dermatologists on test sets of dermoscopy images. These studies provide credibility for pursuing research in this area and the next task is to develop techniques that enable DNNs to become valued clinical decision support tools. We have shown that GradCAM and kernel SHAP maps pass some basic sanity checks and can provide insight into potential sources of bias. However, it is clear that more work is needed before these maps can provide clinically meaningful information. We have also shown that evaluating models according to AUC alone provides limited insight into the true nature of the performance of the model: saliency maps show that models with the same AUC can make predictions using completely different rationales.

Acknowledgement. This work was supported by an Australian Research Council Centre of Excellence for Quantum Engineered Systems grant (CE 110001013).

References

1. Aas, K., Jullum, M., Løland, A.: Explaining individual predictions when features are dependent: more accurate approximations to shapley values. arXiv preprint arXiv:1903.10464 (2019)
2. Adebayo, J., Gilmer, J., Muelly, M., Goodfellow, I., Hardt, M., Kim, B.: Sanity checks for saliency maps. In: Advances in Neural Information Processing Systems, pp. 9505–9515 (2018)
3. Brinker, T.J., et al.: Deep learning outperformed 136 of 157 dermatologists in a head-to-head dermoscopic melanoma image classification task. Eur. J. Cancer **113**, 47–54 (2019)
4. Brinker, T.J., et al.: Skin cancer classification using convolutional neural networks: systematic review. J. Med. Internet Res. **20**(10), e11936 (2018)
5. Chen, J., Song, L., Wainwright, M.J., Jordan, M.I.: L-shapley and C-shapley: efficient model interpretation for structured data. arXiv preprint arXiv:1808.02610 (2018)
6. Elmore, J.G.: Pathologists' diagnosis of invasive melanoma and melanocytic proliferations: observer accuracy and reproducibility study. BMJ **357** (2017). https://doi.org/10.1136/bmj.j2813
7. Esteva, A., et al.: Dermatologist-level classification of skin cancer with deep neural networks. Nature **542**(7639), 115 (2017)
8. Fujisawa, Y., et al.: Deep-learning-based, computer-aided classifier developed with a small dataset of clinical images surpasses board-certified dermatologists in skin tumour diagnosis. Br. J. Dermatol. **180**(2), 373–381 (2019)
9. Haenssle, H., et al.: Man against machine: diagnostic performance of a deep learning convolutional neural network for dermoscopic melanoma recognition in comparison to 58 dermatologists. Ann. Oncol. **29**(8), 1836–1842 (2018)

10. Janda, M., Soyer, H.: Can clinical decision making be enhanced by artificial intelligence? Br. J. Dermatol. **180**(2), 247–248 (2019)
11. Lomas, A., Leonardi-Bee, J., Bath-Hextall, F.: A systematic review of worldwide incidence of nonmelanoma skin cancer. Br. J. Dermatol. **166**(5), 1069–1080 (2012)
12. Lundberg, S.M., Lee, S.I.: A unified approach to interpreting model predictions. In: Advances in Neural Information Processing Systems, pp. 4765–4774 (2017)
13. Mahbod, A., Schaefer, G., Ellinger, I., Ecker, R., Pitiot, A., Wang, C.: Fusing fine-tuned deep features for skin lesion classification. Comput. Med. Imaging Graph. **71**, 19–29 (2019)
14. Mar, V., Soyer, H.: Artificial intelligence for melanoma diagnosis: how can we deliver on the promise? (2018)
15. Molnar, C.: Interpretable Machine Learning - A Guide for Making Black Box Models explainable (2019). christophm.github.io/interpretable-ml-book/
16. Raasch, B.: Suspicious skin lesions and their management. Aust. Fam. Physician **28**(5), 466–471 (1999)
17. Rogers, H.W., et al.: Incidence estimate of nonmelanoma skin cancer in the united states, 2006. Arch. Dermatol. **146**(3), 283–287 (2010)
18. Schadendorf, D., et al.: Melanoma. The Lancet **392**(10151), 971–984 (2018)
19. Selvaraju, R.R., Cogswell, M., Das, A., Vedantam, R., Parikh, D., Batra, D.: Grad-CAM: visual explanations from deep networks via gradient-based localization. In: Proceedings of the IEEE International Conference on Computer Vision, pp. 618–626 (2017)
20. Shapley, L.S.: A value for n-person games. Contrib. Theory Games **2**(28), 307–317 (1953)
21. Simpson, B., Dutil, F., Bengio, Y., Cohen, J.P.: GradMask: reduce overfitting by regularizing saliency. arXiv preprint arXiv:1904.07478 (2019)
22. Tschandl, P., Rosendahl, C., Kittler, H.: The HAM10000 dataset, a large collection of multi-source dermatoscopic images of common pigmented skin lesions. Sci. Data **5**, 180161 (2018)
23. Wang, Z., Bovik, A.C., Sheikh, H.R., Simoncelli, E.P., et al.: Image quality assessment: from error visibility to structural similarity. IEEE Trans. Image Process. **13**(4), 600–612 (2004)

Towards Interpretability of Segmentation Networks by Analyzing DeepDreams

Vincent Couteaux[1,2]([envelope]), Olivier Nempont[2], Guillaume Pizaine[2], and Isabelle Bloch[1]

[1] LTCI, Télécom Paris, Institut polytechnique de Paris, Paris, France
vincent.couteaux@telecom-paristech.fr
[2] Philips Research Paris, Suresnes, France

Abstract. Interpretability of a neural network can be expressed as the identification of patterns or features to which the network can be either sensitive or indifferent. To this aim, a method inspired by DeepDream is proposed, where the activation of a neuron is maximized by performing gradient ascent on an input image. The method outputs curves that show the evolution of features during the maximization. A controlled experiment shows how it enables to assess the robustness to a given feature, or by contrast its sensitivity. The method is illustrated on the task of segmenting tumors in liver CT images.

Keywords: Interpretability · Deep Learning · DeepDream · Segmentation · Liver CT images

1 Introduction

Interpretability of deep neural networks is becoming more and more crucial as deep learning algorithms perform critical tasks such as driving a car or assisting a physician in establishing a diagnosis. In this work we are interested in interpreting segmentation networks by appraising their sensitivity to high-level features. Indeed, segmenting anatomical structures in medical images is one of the tasks that hugely benefited from Convolutional Neural Networks (CNNs), to the point that this framework is now state-of-the-art in most segmentation tasks [5,6,8].

Research on interpretable Deep Learning has been very active for a few years now. Thorough reviews [1,7] extensively describe the field, among which so-called saliency methods are especially popular [4,14,16,17]. The understanding of these methods has grown recently, with some works examining their limitations [11,18]. More generally, saliency methods address the problem of *feature attribution* which, in the case of a segmentation network, boils down to pixel attribution and is thus of limited value.

Another class of interpretability methods consists in visualizing patterns that activate a particular neuron in the network. Most of them consist in maximizing

© Springer Nature Switzerland AG 2019
K. Suzuki et al. (Eds.): ML-CDS 2019/IMIMIC 2019, LNCS 11797, pp. 56–63, 2019.
https://doi.org/10.1007/978-3-030-33850-3_7

the activation in the input space [13,17,19,20]. These visualizations are insightful when the network is trained on natural images, as they generate natural structures and appearances, but they are harder to interpret on medical images.

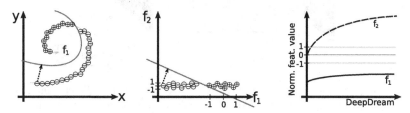

Fig. 1. Illustration of the method with a 2-dimensional classifier. Left: input space, $\oplus$ and $\ominus$ are resp. positive and negative samples; the classification function is the grey line; the data is described by features f_1 (green arrow) and f_2 (orthogonal to f_1). Middle: features space; features are normalized w.r.t. the set of positive samples. Left and middle: the path of steepest slope (or *DeepDream path*) is represented as a dotted arrow. Right: projection of this path on f_1 and f_2 (DeepDream analysis). (Color figure online)

The method in [10] is closer to our motivation, *i.e.* to analyze the influence of human-understandable features on the output of a network. Using abstract concepts defined by sets of example images is appealing, especially for complex concepts that would be difficult to model. But this transfers the burden to the creation of concept-labelled databases, which can be challenging in medical imaging. On the other hand, image domain features such as radiomic features can be used to directly evaluate relevant concepts in medical images when a segmentation mask is available, and seems therefore well suited to the interpretation of segmentation networks.

We detail our method in Sect. 2, starting by giving an intuitive definition of what the *sensitivity* and *robustness* to a feature might be for a network. Then we describe our method based on activation maximization to highlight features that the network is sensitive to (Sect. 2.2). We show in a controlled setting that the method correctly assesses the robustness of a network to a specific feature. Other experiments show how we can get insights about what a network has learned using our method (Sect. 3).

2   Method

2.1   Overview

Segmentation networks achieve state-of-the-art performance on most segmentation tasks. They can extract complex features at multiple scales and successfully perform challenging segmentation tasks where modeling approaches using hand-crafted features would have failed. To interpret this complex decision function, we want to determine how *sensitive* or *robust* a neural network is to a set of

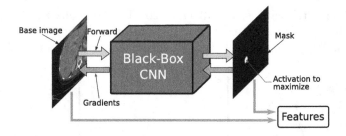

Fig. 2. Representation of an iteration as described in Sect. 2.2: the current image is forwarded in a segmentation CNN. We retrieve the output map and the gradient w.r.t. an arbitrary neuron activation from the output map. We compute the features from the image and segmentation mask and update the image following the gradient for the next iteration.

high-level features $\{f_k\}_{1 \leq k \leq K}$, such as the size of the object, statistics on its intensity distribution or its shape.

We consider that a network is sensitive to a feature f_k if its alteration impacts the network decision. Conversely, we say that the network is robust - or indifferent - to a feature if it is not sensitive to it. However a feature of an object cannot in general be modified without modifying others characteristics, therefore such properties cannot be directly evaluated. Starting from a baseline producing a negative response, we can find a minimal alteration that produces a positive response by following the path of steepest slope in the input space (the arrow in Fig. 1), using the network gradients. This procedure is similar to activation maximization, also known as *DeepDream* [15]. If the features f_k are smooth functions, we can assume that the path of steepest slope in the input space will favor features to which the network is the most sensitive.

In Fig. 1 we provide a schematic view of this process in two dimensions. Intuitively, a network should be indifferent to a feature that is useless (here f_2) for characterizing an object, and sensitive to a feature that is essential (here f_1).

2.2 Algorithm

Being given a trained binary segmentation network S of any architecture, we compute the *DeepDream analysis* with an iterative algorithm, illustrated in Fig. 2. It starts from an image X_0 with no foreground (an image with no lesion in the case of lesion segmentation for instance), and pick a neuron i we want to maximize. At each iteration j and until convergence:

- We forward the image X_j through the network and retrieve the segmentation mask $M_j = S(X_j)$, as well the gradient of the neuron activation $\frac{\partial i}{\partial X}$.
- We update the image for the next iteration $X_{j+1} = X_j + \alpha \frac{\partial i}{\partial X}$.
- We compute features $f_k(X_j, M_j)$.

The output is a plot of the curves $j \rightarrow f_k(X_j, M_j)$. These curves can be interpreted to assess the sensitivity of the network to those features.

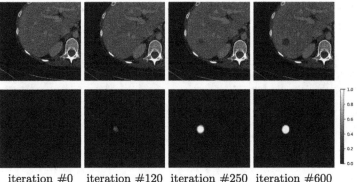

iteration #0   iteration #120   iteration #250   iteration #600

Fig. 3. Different steps of gradient ascent performed on a CT slice showing a healthy liver, with a network trained to segment liver tumors from CT slices. The top row shows the image being "DeepDreamed", while the bottom row shows the output of the network (high probabilities of a pixel being part of a tumor are white, low probabilities are black). The red cross on the leftmost image shows the pixel maximized by gradient ascent. We observe that a responding area appears during the procedure. (Color figure online)

This procedure, derived from activation maximization also known as Deep-Dream, has been shown to work on many classification network architectures [13,17,19,20] and we found that it was easily applicable on several segmentation architectures. Figure 3 shows how the image and segmentation mask respond to the activation maximization.

Although any kind of features can be used, we chose to use radiomic features as they are specifically designed to characterize segmented tissues in medical images [2,9,21], and have shown to capture enough information for Computer-Aided Diagnosis [3,9].

Our DeepDream analysis consists in computing a set of features $f_k(X_j, M_j)$ at each step j of the DeepDream path. As activation maximization produces small changes in input but decisive changes in output, we expect the features to be tweaked according to the sensitivity of the network to those features. To interpret the evolution of feature values observed during the DeepDream analysis, we normalize a particular feature with respect to the distribution of this feature computed on the validation dataset used during training.

3   Experiments

We conduct three experiments to assess the potential of a DeepDream analysis to interpret a segmentation network. We show that the sensitivity computed from the DeepDream analysis is associated with the performance of the network, as expected (Sect. 3.1). The second experiment shows how our method highlights the difference of sensitivities between networks trained on different databases

(Sect. 3.2). Finally we show what kind of insight we can get with our method by applying it to the the real-world use case of liver tumor segmentation (Sect. 3.3).

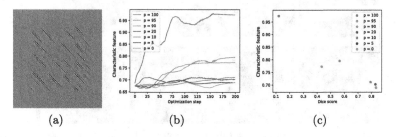

(a)   (b)   (c)

Fig. 4. Controlled experiment. We trained 7 networks with different probabilities p of marking the positively labeled zones. (a) DeepDream of the network for $p = 100\%$. (b) Evolution of the characteristic feature during the gradient ascent process. (c) Dice score on the unmarked test set and characteristic feature at the end of the gradient ascent process for the 7 networks. Networks that performed poorly on the unmarked test set and thus relied on the marking showed a high characteristic feature in their dream.

For all experiments we use basic contracting-expanding architectures with 3×3 convolutions, max-pooling or up-convolution every 2 convolution layers and number of filters doubling at each level, trained with an Adam optimizer until convergence.

3.1   DeepDream Sensitivity and Segmentation Performance

In order to get a setting where the actual sensitivity to a feature is known, we ran the following experiment: For *cat* and *dog* classes from the COCO database [12], each image is augmented with a marking with a probability p. We chose a synthetic texture made of 135° line segments of random positions and intensities as the marking. Then, for different values of p, we train several networks G_p to segment cats and dogs on this training dataset.

A simple, intuitive way to assess the robustness of a network with respect to the marking is then to compute its score on a test dataset with no marking. Given the score of G_0 as the baseline, a similar score indicates that a network is robust to the marking.

We assess the presence of the marking in any DeepDream generated as described in Sect. 2.2 by computing the maximum response of the convolution of the dream with a 135° line segment. We call this feature the *characteristic feature* of the marking. Starting from the same realization of white noise, we then compute the characteristic feature at each optimization step, for all networks G_p. Results are illustrated in Fig. 4.

Networks reaching a Dice score close to the baseline ($p \leq 20\%$) did not see the characteristic feature evolve during DeepDream, in contrast to those which relied on the marking ($p \geq 90\%$). This shows that we are able to correctly assess the sensitivity of a network to a particular feature by analyzing its DeepDreams.

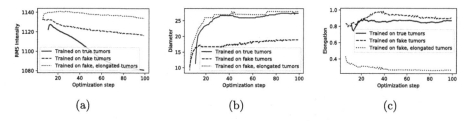

Fig. 5. DeepDream analysis of 3 networks trained on different datasets. (a) Root mean squared intensity along the DeepDream Path. (b) Maximum diameter of the dreamed tumor. (c) Elongation (1 means round, and 0 means elongated in the standard definition of elgontation in radiomics.)

3.2 Sensitivity to Intensity and Shape Features

In the LiTS database[1], tumors appear as hypointense areas in the liver parenchyma. In this experiment we compare a network trained on real tumors to a network trained on synthetic tumors, to test how our method highlights the differences of two networks trained on seemingly similar tasks.

We generate synthetic tumors by lowering the intensities in random areas of healthy livers. The DeepDream analysis shows that the network trained on real tumors is more sensitive to low intensities in the liver (Fig. 5a) than the network trained on synthetic tumors. This indicates that the synthetic network focuses on other features than the intensity.

To determine if the DeepDream analysis is also able to assess the sensitivity to shape features, we train a network to segment only synthetic elongated tumors, as opposed to the overall round shape of real tumors, as observed in clinical environments. We observe that the network trained on elongated tumors is indeed more sensitive to elongation (Fig. 5c).

3.3 Analysis of a Tumor Segmentation Network

To illustrate how one can use DeepDream analysis with radiomic features, we analyze a network trained to segment liver tumors in CT scans. We visualize the evolution of 6 relevant radiomic features, normalized so that 0 is the mean value of the feature computed on the validation dataset, and 1 is one standard deviation above the mean (Fig. 6).

The values of intensity and sphericity quickly evolve towards the normal range, indicating that the network is sensitive to both features. By contrast, the Grey-Level Co-occurrence Matrix (GLCM) Contrast, a texture feature that measures intensity disparity among neighboring pixels, as well as the entropy of the intensities distribution, stay below the normal range, indicating that the network is robust to heterogeneity. This is coherent with our intuition that the network should react to flat hypointense areas in the liver, without significant texture

---

[1] https://competitions.codalab.org/competitions/17094.

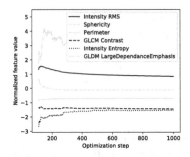

Fig. 6. Evolution of features along the DeepDream path of a liver tumors segmentation network, starting from a healthy liver. Images and masks are shown in Fig. 3.

information. However we also notice that the value of the Large Dependence Emphasis feature goes rapidly and strongly out of normal range, suggesting a lack of robustness to this feature.

4   Conclusion

In this paper, we proposed a new approach to interpret segmentation networks. We generate and analyze fake positive objects using a gradient ascent method. This provides insights on the sensitivity and robustness of the trained network to specific high-level features.

Future work will focus on formulating theoretically grounded definitions of sensitivity and robustness and on providing theoretical guarantees that Deep-Dream primarily modifies the most sensitive features. Other state-of-the-art segmentation architectures (such as U-Nets, DeepLab or PSPNet) will also be tested, as well as multiclass segmentation networks.

References

1. Adadi, A., Berrada, M.: Peeking inside the black-box: a survey on explainable artificial intelligence (XAI). IEEE Access **6**, 52138–52160 (2018)
2. Aerts, H.J.W.L., et al.: Decoding tumour phenotype by noninvasive imaging using a quantitative radiomics approach. Nat. Commun. **5**, 4006 (2014)
3. Avanzo, M., Stancanello, J., Naqa, I.M.E.: Beyond imaging: the promise of radiomics. Phys. Med. Eur. J. Med. Phys. **38**, 122–139 (2017)
4. Bach, S., et al.: On pixel-wise explanations for non-linear classifier decisions by layer-wise relevance propagation. PloS ONE **10**(7), e0130140 (2015)
5. Christ, P.F., et al.: Automatic liver and tumor segmentation of CT and MRI volumes using cascaded fully convolutional neural networks. CoRR abs/1702.05970 (2017)
6. Couteaux, V., et al.: Kidney cortex segmentation in 2D CT with U-Nets ensemble aggregation. Diagn. Intervent. Imaging **100**, 211–217 (2019)
7. Doshi-Velez, F., Kim, B.: Towards a rigorous science of interpretable machine learning. arXiv preprint arXiv:1702.08608 (2017)

8. Erden, B., Gamboa, N., Wood, S.: 3D convolutional neural network for brain tumor segmentation. Computer Science, Stanford University, USA, Technical report (2017)

9. Gillies, R.J., Kinahan, P.E., Hricak, H.: Radiomics: images are more than pictures, they are data. Radiology **278**(2), 563–577 (2015)

10. Kim, B., et al.: Interpretability beyond feature attribution: quantitative testing with concept activation vectors (TCAV). In: ICML (2018)

11. Kindermans, P.J., et al.: The (un) reliability of saliency methods. arXiv preprint arXiv:1711.00867 (2017)

12. Lin, T.-Y., et al.: Microsoft COCO: common objects in context. In: Fleet, D., Pajdla, T., Schiele, B., Tuytelaars, T. (eds.) ECCV 2014. LNCS, vol. 8693, pp. 740–755. Springer, Cham (2014). https://doi.org/10.1007/978-3-319-10602-1_48

13. Mahendran, A., Vedaldi, A.: Visualizing deep convolutional neural networks using natural pre-images. Int. J. Comput. Vision **120**(3), 233–255 (2016)

14. Montavon, G., Lapuschkin, S., Binder, A., Samek, W., Müller, K.R.: Explaining nonlinear classification decisions with deep taylor decomposition. Pattern Recogn. **65**, 211–222 (2017)

15. Mordvintsev, A., Olah, C., Tyka, M.: Inceptionism: Going deeper into neural networks. Google Research Blog (2015)

16. Ribeiro, M.T., Singh, S., Guestrin, C.: "Why Should I Trust You?": explaining the predictions of any classifier. In: HLT-NAACL Demos (2016)

17. Simonyan, K., Vedaldi, A., Zisserman, A.: Deep inside convolutional networks: visualising image classification models and saliency maps. arXiv preprint arXiv:1312.6034 (2013)

18. Yeh, C.K., Hsieh, C.Y., Suggala, A.S., Inouye, D., Ravikumar, P.: How sensitive are sensitivity-based explanations? arXiv preprint arXiv:1901.09392 (2019)

19. Yosinski, J., Clune, J., Nguyen, A., Fuchs, T., Lipson, H.: Understanding neural networks through deep visualization. arXiv preprint arXiv:1506.06579 (2015)

20. Zeiler, M.D., Fergus, R.: Visualizing and understanding convolutional networks. In: Fleet, D., Pajdla, T., Schiele, B., Tuytelaars, T. (eds.) ECCV 2014. LNCS, vol. 8689, pp. 818–833. Springer, Cham (2014). https://doi.org/10.1007/978-3-319-10590-1_53

21. Zwanenburg, A., Leger, S., Vallières, M., Löck, S., et al.: Image biomarker standardisation initiative. arXiv preprint arXiv:1612.07003 (2016)

9th International Workshop on Multimodal Learning for Clinical Decision Support (ML-CDS 2019)

Towards Automatic Diagnosis
from Multi-modal Medical Data

Jiang Tian[✉], Cheng Zhong, Zhongchao Shi, and Feiyu Xu

AI Lab, Lenovo Research, Beijing, China
{tianjiang1,zhongcheng3,shizc2,fxu}@lenovo.com

Abstract. Many healthcare applications would significantly benefit from the processing and analyzing of multi-modal data. In this paper, we propose a novel multi-task, multi-modal, and multi-attention framework to learn and align information from multiple medical sources. Based on experiments on a public medical dataset, we show that combining features from images (e.g. x-rays) and texts (e.g. clinical reports), sharing information among different tasks (e.g. x-rays classification, autoencoder, and diagnosis generation) and across domains boost the performance of diagnosis generation (86.0% in terms of BLEU@4).

1 Introduction

In healthcare, there have been continuous efforts and progresses in the automatic recognition and localization of specific diseases and organs, mostly on radiology images. Meanwhile, recent image/video captioning techniques [1,2] by deep learning enable the generation of a description about the content of a medical image automatically like a report written by a human radiologist [3,4], which have a big impact for countries like China where doctors have a very big work load, and has vast potentials to renovate medical computer-aided diagnosis (CAD).

On the other hand, in healthcare, different types of information are available from different sources such as electronic health care records, patient summaries, clinical test results, and imaging (e.g. x-rays, CT scans, etc.). This data can be both structured and unstructured. Vast amount of information is currently held in medical records in the form of free text. The fusion of healthcare data from multiple sources could take advantage of existing synergies between data to improve clinical decisions and to reveal entirely new approaches to treating diseases.

Inspired by this fact, in order to learn and relate information from multiple sources and identify implicit correlations not visible when considering only one source of data, we build a multi-task, multi-modal, and multi-attention framework in this paper. It treats the generation on diagnosis as a text generation task, where the encoded information is from chest x-rays, patient's indication, and doctor's observations of the image. We use a publicly available radiology dataset of chest x-rays and reports [5]. The dataset contains 7,470 pairs of x-ray and report.

© Springer Nature Switzerland AG 2019
K. Suzuki et al. (Eds.): ML-CDS 2019/IMIMIC 2019, LNCS 11797, pp. 67–74, 2019.
https://doi.org/10.1007/978-3-030-33850-3_8

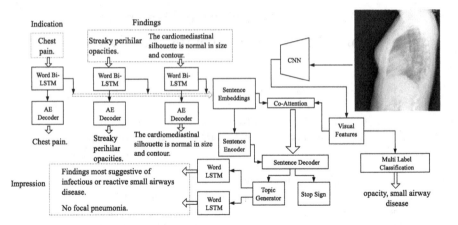

Fig. 1. Overall illustration of the proposed multi-task, multi-modal, and multi-attention framework. An LSTM model is utilized to hierarchically build embeddings for a paragraph from embeddings for sentences and words. Combined with the joint visual and textual attention mechanism, another hierarchical LSTM first generates topics, and then decodes this embedding to generate sentences for diagnosis. This hierarchical encoder-decoder is co-opted by a second neural autoencoder (AE) for the input sentences. The AE shares the same bidirectional LSTM (BiLSTM) for words.

Each report consists of the following sections: *indication*, *findings*, *tags*, and *impression*, in line with a common radiology reporting format for diagnostic chest x-rays study. The *indication* section is a simple, concise statement of the reason for the study. The *findings* section of the report includes the description of the results of the study. The *tags* section lists the keywords which represent the critical information in the *findings*. In a radiology report, the summary has been referred to as the *impression, conclusion, or diagnosis* section. Most physicians read only the *impression* section of a radiology report, which places great importance on this section of the report.

As shown in Fig. 1, our model takes an x-ray, and multiple sentences describing *indication* and *findings* as input, generates textual descriptions of *impression*. The use of appropriate recommendations in the *impression* section can greatly contribute to the management of patient care and can provide consultative information that may not otherwise be available. The framework is designed to take advantage of the compositional structure of both visual and textual information.

2   Model

Our work draws on recent progresses in LSTM auto-encoder to preserve and reconstruct multi-sentence paragraphs [6], hierarchical attention network for document classification [7], and multi-task learning [8] and its application for video encoder and language entailment generation [9].

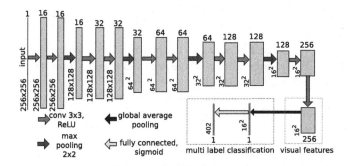

Fig. 2. Visual encoder architecture (best viewed in color). The number of channels is denoted either on top of or below the box. The x-y size is provided at the lower left edge of the box. (Color figure online)

2.1 X-ray Encoding and Multi Label Classification

The architecture of x-rays encoder is illustrated in Fig. 2. Visual features in Fig. 2 denote conv-feature maps with dimension $256 \times (16 \times 16)$ generated by the image model. It has two branches, one for predicting x-ray image tags, and another for visual context for the text generation model.

We treat the tag prediction task as a multi-label classification (MLC). Specifically, a fully connected layer and a sigmoid one are adopted after global average pooling of the visual features, which generates a distribution over all of the tags.

The x-ray encoder compresses the visual information into a 16×16 feature map, where each pixel has a 256-dimensional feature vector. The attention module in Sect. 2.3 performs spatial attention over this feature map.

2.2 Hierarchical Textual Encoder and Decoder

Throughout the paper, we will denote by $LSTM(\mathbf{h}_{t-1}, \mathbf{y}_t)$ the LSTM operation on vectors $\mathbf{h}_{t-1}$ and $\mathbf{y}_t$ to achieve $\mathbf{h}_t$. $\mathbf{h}_t^w$ and $\mathbf{h}_t^s$ denote hidden states from LSTMs, the superscripts of which denote operation at word level w or sentence level s, the subscripts of which indicate time step t. $\mathbf{h}_t^w(en)$ specifies encoding stage and $\mathbf{h}_t^w(de)$ implies decoding one. $\mathbf{y}_t^w$ and $\mathbf{y}_t^s$ denote word level and sentence level embedding at time t.

We first obtain representation at the sentence level by running one BiLSTM on top of its containing words.

$$\mathbf{h}_t^w(en) = BiLSTM_{en}^w(\mathbf{h}_{t-1}^w(en), \mathbf{y}_t^w(en)). \tag{1}$$

The output at the ending time step is used to represent the entire sentence as $\mathbf{y}_s = \mathbf{h}_{end_s}^w$.

To build representation for the whole paragraph, another layer of LSTM is placed on top of all sentences, computing sequentially for each time step as

$$\mathbf{h}_t^s(en) = LSTM_{en}^s(\mathbf{h}_{t-1}^s(en), \mathbf{y}_t^s(en)). \tag{2}$$

Representation computed at the final time step is used to represent the entire paragraph $\mathbf{y}_p = \mathbf{h}^s_{end_p}$.

Furthermore, one BiLSTM operates at the word level, which leads to sentence representations. These embedding vectors are then used as inputs into the LSTM which acquires paragraph representation.

Similar to encoding, the decoding module operates on a hierarchical structure with two layers of LSTMs. LSTM outputs at sentence level for time step t are obtained by:

$$\mathbf{h}^s_t(de) = LSTM^s_{de}(\mathbf{h}^s_{t-1}(de), \mathbf{y}^s_t(de), \mathbf{z}_t), \tag{3}$$

where $\mathbf{z}_t$ is a context vector, which will be explained in detail in Sect. 2.3. It allows for salient features to dynamically come to the forefront as needed. The initial time step $\mathbf{h}^s_0(de)$ is equal to $\mathbf{y}_p$, the output from the encoding procedure.

We use a deep output layer [10] to generate topic vector as follows.

$$\mathbf{t}^s = relu(G_{t1}(relu(G_{t0}\mathbf{h}^s_t(de)))), \tag{4}$$

where G_{t0} and G_{t1} are parameter matrices. $\mathbf{t}^s$ is used as the initial input into $LSTM^w_{de}$ for subsequently predicting words sequentially within sentence $t + 1$. The prediction stops when #end, which designates the end of a sentence, is emitted. The process is summarized as follows.

$$\mathbf{h}^w_t(de) = LSTM^w_{de}(\mathbf{h}^w_{t-1}(de), \mathbf{y}^w_t(de)), \tag{5}$$

$$p(w|\mathbf{h}^w_t(de)) \propto exp(\mathbf{h}^w_t(de), \mathbf{y}^w_t(de)). \tag{6}$$

During decoding, the hidden state of $LSTM^w_{de}$ computed at the final time step is used to represent the current sentence, which is passed to $LSTM^s_{de}$, combined with $\mathbf{h}^s_t(de)$ for the acquisition of $\mathbf{h}^s_{t+1}(de)$, and outputted to the next time step in sentence decoding.

For each time step t, $LSTM^s_{de}$ has to first decide whether decoding should proceed or come to a stop. A linear projection from $\mathbf{h}^s_t(de)$ and a logistic classifier produce a distribution over $[STOP = 1, CONTINUE = 0]$ as

$$p(stop|\mathbf{h}^s_t(de)) \propto exp(G_{stop}\mathbf{h}^s_t(de) + B_{stop}), \tag{7}$$

where G_{stop} and B_{stop} are parameter matrices. If $p(stop|\mathbf{h}^s_t(de))$ is greater than a predefined threshold (e.g. 0.5), then $LSTM^s_{de}$ will stop producing new topic vectors and $LSTM^w_{de}$ will also stop producing words.

At the same time, we utilize the $one - to - many$ approach [9] for tasks that have an encoder in common. A separate decoder (AE Decoder in Fig. 1) is used to generate the same sequence of words, which reconstructs the inputs, vector representations from the aforementioned $BiLSTM^w_{en}$, by predicting words within sentences sequentially from an $LSTM^{ae}_{de}$.

2.3   Joint Textual and Visual Attention

Indication and *findings* in a report are encoded into a set of vectors as $d = \{\mathbf{d}_0, \cdots, \mathbf{d}_{\Pi-1}\}$, where Π is the total number of sentences.

A textual context vector $\mathbf{z}_d = \sum_{i=0}^{\Pi-1} \alpha_{ti}\mathbf{d}_i$ is a dynamic vector that represents the relevant part of textual feature at time step t, where α_{ti} is a scalar weighting of textual vector $\mathbf{d}_i$ at time step t, defined as follows.

$$\alpha_{ti} = exp(e_{ti})/\sum_{k=0}^{\Pi-1} exp(e_{tk}), \qquad e_{ti} = f_{att}(\mathbf{d}_i, \mathbf{h}_t^s(de)), \qquad (8)$$

where f_{att} is a function that determines the amount of attention allocated to textual feature $\mathbf{d}_i$, conditioned on the LSTM hidden state $\mathbf{h}_t^s(de)$. This function is implemented as a multilayer perceptron as $f_{att} = \mathbf{w}^T tanh(U_d\mathbf{h}_t^s(de) + W_d\mathbf{d}_i + \mathbf{b}_d)$. Note that by construction $\sum_{i=0}^{\Pi-1} \alpha_{ti} = 1$.

The visual encoder network encodes an x-ray image into a set of vectors as $a = \{\mathbf{a}_0, \cdots, \mathbf{a}_{255}\}$. Similarly, we can construct a visual context vector $\mathbf{z}_a$. Finally, we combine the textual and visual context vectors using concatenation as $\mathbf{z}_t = [\mathbf{z}_d, \mathbf{z}_a]$.

3 Experiments

Among the $7,470$ pairs of image and report, there are $6,461$ cases which have both *findings* and *impression* in the report. We randomly select 500 samples for validation and 500 cases for testing. Training is conducted on the remaining $5,461$ ones.

We preprocess the data through converting all tokens to lower cases, and removing all of non-alpha tokens. It leads to 401 unique tags, each of which appears at least twice, covering 96.0% tag occurrences in the dataset, and 1331 unique words, each of which appears at least three times in all sentences, covering 99.0% word occurrences in the dataset. The uncovered tags and words are replaced with a special *UNK* token. On average, each x-ray image is associated with 2.2 tags, 1.7, 4.7, 1.4 sentences for *indication*, *findings*, and *impression*, respectively. The x-ray images are resized to a size of 256×256.

An illustration of diagnosis generation by our model is shown in Fig. 5. In our experiments, the hidden state size from all LSTMs is empirically set to 512 as it has a better tradeoff between performance and model complexity. We evaluate the diagnosis generation performance on the BLEU(B) [11] and ROUGE(R) [12] scores over all of the testing reports.

The results are given in Table 1. The first row (MTMA) lists results of our major model defined in Fig. 1. The second row (MTMA-AE) presents a model (Fig. 3) without adding AE Decoder to the BiLSTM encoder in the major model. The third row (MTMA-IM) lists results from a configuration (Fig. 4) where diagnosis is from *indication* and *findings* only. The fourth row (Jing) shows results from an x-ray captioning [13] for the same dataset as we use, wherein, a hierarchical LSTM model is utilized to generate a paragraph on the contents in *impression* and *findings* from encoding of the x-ray. By adding auxiliary task connected to the encoder, we would expect to encourage encoder in the lower

Table 1. BLEU@n and ROUGE scores on diagnosis generation. All values are reported as percentage (%).

Method	B1	B2	B3	B4	R
MTMA	88.2	87.4	86.7	86.0	92.9
MTMA-AE	55.8	51.6	47.6	43.2	82.2
MTMA-IM	52.1	48.1	44.1	39.8	82.2
Jing	51.7	38.6	30.6	24.7	44.7

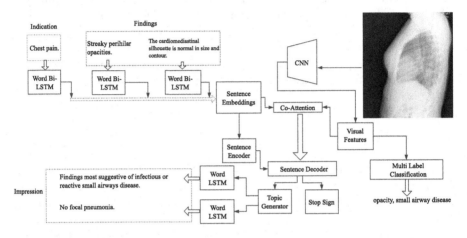

Fig. 3. Illustration of the proposed multi-task, multi-modal, and multi-attention framework without neural autoencoder (AE) for the input sentences. An LSTM model is utilized to hierarchically build embeddings for a paragraph from embeddings for sentences and words. Combined with the joint visual and textual attention mechanism, another hierarchical LSTM first generates topics, and then decodes this embedding to generate sentences for diagnosis.

stages provides additional regularization and better generalization. The comparison between MTMA and MTMA-AE indicates that by training on another relatively small task jointly, the model improves its performance on its main task. Employing joint visual and textual information for generating topics does help diagnosis generation a lot by comparison between MTMA with MTMA-IM and Jing. The reason might be that visual attention can capture sub-region image information, and textual attention focuses on semantic context, which is confirmed by visual input. It suggests that our framework provides better alignment from *impression* output to the provided visual and textual features. In summary, MTMA achieves the best results on all of the evaluation metrics, which demonstrates the effectiveness of the proposed multi-task, multi-attention model using multi-modal data fusion.

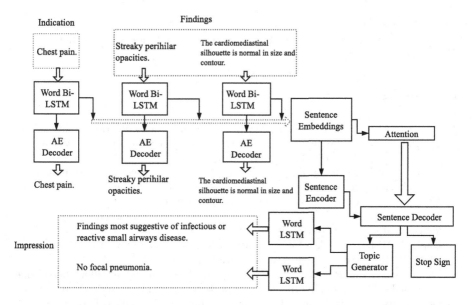

Fig. 4. Illustration of the proposed multi-task framework without x-ray input. An LSTM model is utilized to hierarchically build embeddings for a paragraph from embeddings for sentences and words. With textual attention mechanism, another hierarchical LSTM first generates topics, and then decodes this embedding to generate sentences for diagnosis.

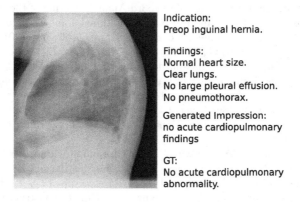

Fig. 5. Illustration of diagnosis generated by the model defined in Fig. 1. GT represents ground truth *impression* from the report.

4   Conclusion

This paper proposes a multi-task, multi-modal, and multi-attention framework to learn and align medical information from multiple sources. Due to different types of information available from different sources in healthcare, it has a big impact for CAD. Through experiments on a publicly available radiology dataset of chest x-rays and reports, we show that combining features from images and text can improve the performance of diagnosis generation (86.0% in terms of BLEU@4).

References

1. Xu, J., Mei, T., Yao, T., Rui, Y.: MSR-VTT: a large video description dataset for bridging video and language. In: 2016 IEEE Conference on Computer Vision and Pattern Recognition, pp. 5288–5296 (2016)
2. Yu, H., Wang, J., Huang, Z., Yang, Y., Xu, W.: Video paragraph captioning using hierarchical recurrent neural networks. In: 2016 IEEE Conference on Computer Vision and Pattern Recognition, pp. 4584–4593 (2016)
3. Xu, T., Zhang, H., Huang, X., Zhang, S., Metaxas, D.N.: Multimodal deep learning for cervical dysplasia diagnosis. In: Ourselin, S., Joskowicz, L., Sabuncu, M.R., Unal, G., Wells, W. (eds.) MICCAI 2016. LNCS, vol. 9901, pp. 115–123. Springer, Cham (2016). https://doi.org/10.1007/978-3-319-46723-8_14
4. Zhang, Z., Chen, P., Sapkota, M., Yang, L.: TandemNet: distilling knowledge from medical images using diagnostic reports as optional semantic references. In: Descoteaux, M., Maier-Hein, L., Franz, A., Jannin, P., Collins, D.L., Duchesne, S. (eds.) MICCAI 2017. LNCS, vol. 10435, pp. 320–328. Springer, Cham (2017). https://doi.org/10.1007/978-3-319-66179-7_37
5. Demner-Fushman, D., et al.: Preparing a collection of radiology examinations for distribution and retrieval. J. Am. Med. Inform. Assoc. **23**(2), 304–310 (2016)
6. Li, J., Luong, T., Jurafsky, D.: A hierarchical neural autoencoder for paragraphs and documents. In: Proceedings of the 53rd Annual Meeting of the Association for Computational Linguistics and the 7th International Joint Conference on Natural Language Processing (Volume 1: Long Papers), pp. 1106–1115 (2015)
7. Yang, Z., Yang, D., Dyer, C., He, X., Smola, A.J., Hovy, E.H.: Hierarchical attention networks for document classification. In: Proceedings of the 2016 Conference of the North American Chapter of the Association for Computational Linguistics: Human Language Technologies, pp. 1480–1489 (2016)
8. Luong, M.T., Le, Q.V., Sutskever, I., Vinyals, O., Kaiser, L.: Multi-task sequence to sequence learning. In: International Conference on Learning Representations 2016, May 2016
9. Pasunuru, R., Bansal, M.: Multi-task video captioning with video and entailment generation. In: Proceedings of the 55th Annual Meeting of the Association for Computational Linguistics (Volume 1: Long Papers), pp. 1273–1283 (2017)
10. Pascanu, R., Gülçehre, Ç., Cho, K., Bengio, Y.: How to construct deep recurrent neural networks. In: International Conference on Learning Representations 2014 (2014)
11. Papineni, K., Roukos, S., Ward, T., Zhu, W.J.: BLEU: a method for automatic evaluation of machine translation. In: Proceedings of 40th Annual Meeting of the Association for Computational Linguistics, pp. 311–318 (2002)
12. Lin, C.Y.: Rouge: a package for automatic evaluation of summaries. In: Text Summarization Branches Out: Proceedings of the ACL-04 Workshop, pp. 74–81 (2004)
13. Jing, B., Xie, P., Xing, E.P.: On the automatic generation of medical imaging reports. CoRR abs/1711.08195 (2017)

Deep Learning Based Multi-modal Registration for Retinal Imaging

Mustafa Arikan[1,2], Amir Sadeghipour[1,2], Bianca Gerendas[1,2], Reinhard Told[2], and Ursula Schmidt-Erfurt[1,2(✉)]

[1] Christian Doppler Laboratory for Ophthalmic Image Analysis,
Department of Ophthalmology and Optometry,
Medical University of Vienna, Vienna, Austria
`ursula.schmidt-erfurth@meduniwien.ac.at`
[2] Department of Ophthalmology and Optometry,
Medical University of Vienna, Vienna, Austria

Abstract. The precise alignment of retina images from different modalities allows ophthalmologists not only to track morphological/pathological changes over time but also to combine different modalities to approach the diagnosis, prognostication, management and monitoring of a retinal disease. We propose an image registration algorithm to trace changes in the retina structure across modalities using vessel segmentation and automatic landmark detection. The segmentation of the vessels is done using a U-Net and the detection of the vessel junctions is achieved with Mask R-CNN. We evaluated the results of our approach using manual grading by expert readers. In the largest dataset (FA-to-SLO/OCT) containing 1130 pairs we achieve an average error rate of 13.12%. We compared our method with intensity based affine registration methods using original and vessel segmentation images.

1 Introduction

From a clinical perspective there is a need for observing retinal features and pathologies across different imaging modalities for the patient's diagnosis and treatment [11]. Some structures and pathologies are better recognized in a particular modality than in other modalities. In retinal imaging, two common categories of imaging procedures are present. These are 2D imaging methods like *CF* (color fundus photography), *FA* (fluorescein angiography), *FAF* (fundus autofluorescence), *ICGA* (indocyanine green angiography) or *SLO* (scanning laser ophthalmoscopy) and 3D methods like *SD-OCT* (spectral domain optical coherence tomography) or *OCT-A* (optical coherence tomography angiography). 2D methods provide two-dimensional information of the human retina by means of reflected light. OCT and OCT-A provide three-dimensional information of retinal structures such as intraretinal layers and optic nerve head that are not available via e.g. fundus imaging [10]. For example, the fovea position is easier to find in 3D OCT images comparing to 2D modalities such as CF. Using multimodal registration, the fovea position can be annotated in OCT and precisely

© Springer Nature Switzerland AG 2019
K. Suzuki et al. (Eds.): ML-CDS 2019/IMIMIC 2019, LNCS 11797, pp. 75–82, 2019.
https://doi.org/10.1007/978-3-030-33850-3_9

transferred to other modalities. The distinct appearance of retinal structures when imaged with different techniques and the increasing number of scans makes the manual annotation for registration a challenging and time-consuming task. Therefore automatic multi-modal image registration would be beneficial. The goal is to warp a moving image to the coordinate frame of a reference image so that the same point is visualized at the same coordinates in both modalities. The topic of multi-modal image registration has been addressed by a few studies which relied on descriptor matching [7] and feature-based registration [6,10], hough transform [17] or domain-specific landmarks [2].

Recently, convolutional neural networks (CNNs), have shown impressive performance in both image segmentation [14] and detection tasks [1], and have found good applications [3,5,8,15] in retinal imaging. Coupled with these improvements we introduce a multi-modal registration algorithm. To sufficiently tackle the challenge of multi-modal registration in retinal imaging over many different modalities and vendors, vessel segmentation and finding of landmarks is crucial.

In this paper, we propose a novel framework to address the challenging task of automatic multi-modal retinal 2D/3D image registration. The proposed framework is superior to reference intensity based multi-modal registration methods in terms of accuracy and robustness. Specifically, our approach is not limited to a particular pair of modalities and utilizes deep learning for modality-specific segmentation of vessels and detection of vessel junctions. We use vessel segmentations and corresponding vessel junctions for a two-step registration approach, where we first estimate scaling, rotation and translation using landmarks and fine tuning using the vessel segmentation.

In summary, the main contributions of our approach include: high diversity/variety of modalities, robustness against low-quality images where vessels are not captured well, and robust registration. This paper is organized as follows. Section 2 introduces the proposed method. Section 3 describes experiments and the evaluation. Finally, Sect. 4 presents our conclusion and future work.

2   Method

Figure 1 shows the pipeline of the proposed registration framework. The segmentation part is a U-Net [14] based network consisting of 11 layers, i.e., 6 convolutional layers, 2 max-pooling layers, 2 upsampling layers and 1 softmax layer. The training is performed on patches, which are extracted from the training images with certain patch size. We trained five segmentation models for each modality with its own configuration regarding number of epochs, patch height, patch width, batch size and number of training samples. We collected between 12 and 15 image annotations - vessels and markers - for each modality for the training. We extended the number of training samples using data augmentation. We have - while taking account the different image resolutions - generated between 75 and 500 training samples for every modality.

The detection part is a Mask R-CNN [1] (regional CNN) based network for finding automatic landmarks (bifurcations, branches and crossover). The detection part is trained for every modality on the same images as the segmentation part. Mask R-CNN is a network architecture aimed at finding instances of objects in images. In our case we find vessel bifurcations, branches and crossover. We rely on Mask R-CNN instead of ridge detection algorithms, thus we can train modality-specific models for detection and don't need parameter tuning for such methods. The output of our detection models is a bounding box of found objects and a mask representing the instance.

Our main method uses both (segmentation and detection) parts for the registration. We estimate scaling, rotation and translation using sets of points found by the detection part. This is the initial registration between two images. In the final part of the registration we use the vessel segmentations and apply affine registration to do fine-tuning and finish the task of registration.

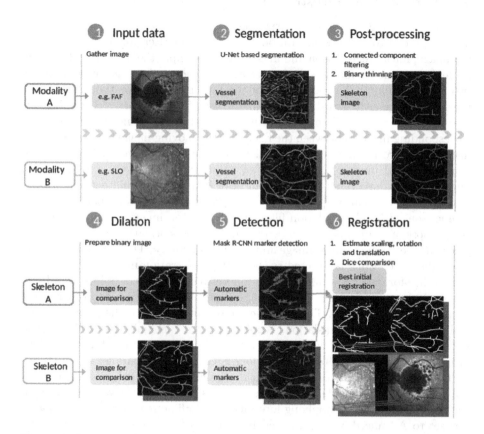

Fig. 1. Architecture of the proposed multi-modal registration pipeline, with the U-Net based segmentation part (1–3), preparation of comparison images (4), the detection part (5) based on Mask R-CNN for automatic markers and registration (6). The registration flow for a pair of scans including segmentation of vessels, finding automatic markers and the step for the initial registration using markers and dice comparison are indicated.

2.1 Segmentation

The segmentation related parts of the pipeline consist of a U-Net based segmentation, a connected component filtering and binary thinning. After the segmentation we apply a connected component filter to remove noise and some vessels, which are isolated and less connected than others. This is done as following: apply Otsu's method [12] on segmentation result, assign a label to every region in the binary image, count the number of pixels for every region, keep the largest N (N = 10) regions and filter the rest of the regions. After the connected component filter, we apply binary thinning to obtain a skeleton of the vessels.

2.2 Detection and Registration

The detection and registration parts consist of a Mask R-CNN to detect automatic markers from the segmentation result, dilation filter applied on the skeleton image, initial registration and fine-tuning. We apply the detection algorithm to detect automatic markers (bifurcations, branches and crossover) and create two lists containing the coordinates of the found markers for the moving and the fixed image. Afterwards, we compile a list of M (e.g. M = 6) neighbours for every marker. For the purpose of initial registration we need at least three corresponding markers between the fixed and the moving image to correctly estimate scaling, rotation and translation. We iterate through every marker and its neighbours and prepare a list of sets of points with size K (K = 3) for both images. Using these sets of points from both images we estimate scaling, rotation and the translation parameters. The skeleton image is prepared for dice comparison: we apply a dilation filter on the skeleton image to gain images for the purpose of comparison. After estimating the transformation we calculate the dice value between the fixed image and the moving image. The combination with the highest dice value is selected as the initial registration matrix. The calculation of dice for every possible combination between the sets of points from both images is computationally expensive. The estimation part on the other hand is computed much faster. Therefore we apply constraints for the parameters of scaling, rotation and translation. For example we can limit the scaling factor between 0.5 and 1.5 and calculate dice for only a subset of combinations. The dice comparison for possible combinations is calculated in parallel to save time. At the end, the combination which yields the highest dice value is selected for the initial registration. The initial registration is used along the vessel images for the final registration by applying intensity based affine registration. The metric was set to Advanced Mattes Mutual Information [9] to measure the similarity of the registration.

Implementation Details: Our registration framework was implemented in Python. We implemented the segmentation network in Keras. The learning rate was initialized as 0.1. The training took between 6 and 9 h for the different modalities. The marker detection (Mask R-CNN) is implemented in Python3 and Caffe. The training took between 12 and 17 h. The networks were trained using a GPU of NVIDIA 1080Ti. The estimation of scaling, rotation and translation is done using nudged [13] (https://github.com/axelpale/nudged). The intensity based affine registration is achieved using the elastix [4] framework (http://elastix.isi.uu.nl/).

3   Experiments

We applied our registration framework on several modalities and data sets. To be able to compare we used the elastix as a reference. We applied our algorithm on FA, FAF, SLO/OCT, ICGA and OCT-A images. We registered pairs of FAF and SLO/OCT images with 1130 examples. The data was acquired at the Ophthalmology Department of the Medical University of Vienna. We also registered ICGA and FA with OCT-A images containing 25 examples. We compared our algorithm with intensity based affine registrations from elastix. The overview of the use cases can be seen in Table 1.

Registration Results. Figure 2 presents the registration results of our proposed framework for a selected example (FAF-to-SLO).

Table 1. Overview of the data sets

Moving image	Fixed image	# of pairs	Remarks
FAF	SLO/OCT	1130	2D-to-2D/3D
FA	OCT-A	25	2D-to-2D/3D
ICGA	FA	25	2D-to-2D

3.1   FAF-to-SLO Registration

SLO is a non-invasive 2D technique to obtain high resolution en face images of the retina. FAF is a non-invasive 2D technique, where vessels are characterized by a reduced signal due to the absorption by blood [16].

We prepared a data set with 1130 pairs from 71 patients with FAF and SLO/OCT images. We registered FAF images (moving image) to SLO images (fixed image). Both the SLO and the FAF images have resolutions of 768×768 or 1536×1536 pixels. The SLO images were scanned together with the OCT and therefore they were already co-registered. Thus in addition to FAF-to-SLO registration we also achieved FAF-to-OCT registration. The registrations were manually evaluated and compared to a reference intensity based affine registration [4]. For the manual evaluation we prepared checkerboard visualizations of registration pairs. We visualized before and after images. The results were evaluated by four expert readers, who looked at every result of the 1130 image pairs. The results of the evaluation were: 13.72%, 12.92%, 12.83% and 13.01% using our method and 30.71%, 28.94%, 30.8% and 32.74% using the reference method. We achieved an average error rate of 13.12% vs. 30.8% using the reference method.

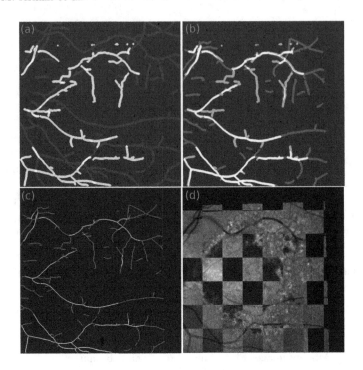

Fig. 2. Registration result of our proposed multi-modal registration framework for FAF-to-SLO/OCT. (a) Overlay visualization before registration of SLO (bright) and FAF (dark). (b) Result of initial registration using Mask R-CNN for automatic markers. (c) Result of affine registration for fine-tuning using vessel segmentations. (d) Transformation applied on original2 images and checkerboard visualization of both.

3.2   FA-to-OCT-A Registration

OCT and OCT-A are non-invasive 3D imaging techniques, that obtain projections of the retinal layers using low-coherence light waves. OCT-A utilizes motion-contrast imaging, calculating differences in backscattered OCT signal intensity between sequential scans of the same area. We used 25 FA images and OCT-A volumes. The FA images have a resolution of 1536×1536 pixels while the OCT-A slabs - projections on a 2D plane of an OCT-A volume between two selected retinal layers - have a resolution of 500×500. The OCT-A slabs cover a smaller area in the 2D plane than the FA images. We registered FA images (moving image) to OCT-A slabs images (fixed image). The registration for images with different resolutions and areas of interest is much more difficult using intensity based affine registrations. We registered 21 out 25 image pairs (error rate 16%) using our method with using ten neighbour landmarks ($M = 10$). We show in Fig. 3 the result of such a registration with different resolutions and sizes using our method. We also highlight the set of points with the best dice from the initial registration.

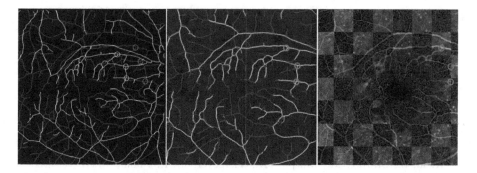

Fig. 3. Registration result for images with different resolutions and sizes for FA-to-OCT-A slab. From left to right: Overlay visualization before registration of FA (bright) and resized OCT-A slab (dark), end result of registration and transformation applied on original images and checkerboard visualization of both. In all three images we highlight the sets of points resulting from our landmark detection and matching algorithm.

3.3   ICGA-to-FA Registration

We used 25 ICGA images and FA images. ICGA is a invasive 2D imaging technique like FA. In ICGA, retinal vasculature is also visualized and it normally appears as a vascular network overlying the choroidal vessels. The ICGA images have the same resolution of 1536×1536 pixels like the FA images. The ICGA images cover a similar area as the FA images. We registered ICGA images (moving) to FA images (fixed). After the registration of ICGA to FA and FA to OCT-A we indirectly registered ICGA to the OCT-A slabs and volumes as well.

4   Conclusion and Future Work

We proposed a novel framework for multi-modal registration of retinal images using vessel segmentation and landmark detection. Intensity based registration methods often fail when images have different resolutions, sizes or grey value ranges. We relied on landmarks, vessels and a matching strategy to overcome the limitations of intensity based affine registration methods. The proposed framework can deal with different image modalities and resolutions. Finally, we applied our method on different combinations of modalities and compared to a intensity based affine registration method. The benefits of automatic landmarks and matching strategies for registration is crucial for noisy and incomplete images. A robust multi-modal registration will help medical doctors to include multiple imaging modalities for disease diagnosis, progression and therapy. Therefore we would like to apply our method on more data and more combinations of retinal imaging modalities. This work constitutes a step towards constructing more robust image registration methods for the high number of different modalities, vendors and image resolutions in retinal imaging. We would like to investigate registration errors using a quantitative evaluation with different number of neighbour markers and the applicability to other medical imaging domains.

References

1. He, K., Gkioxari, G., Dollár, P., Girshick, R.B.: Mask R-CNN. CoRR abs/1703.06870 (2017). http://arxiv.org/abs/1703.06870
2. Hervella, Á.S., Rouco, J., Novo, J., Ortega, M.: Multimodal registration of retinal images using domain-specific landmarks and vessel enhancement. CoRR abs/1803.00951 (2018). http://arxiv.org/abs/1803.00951
3. Khojasteh, P., Aliahmad, B., Kumar, D.K.: Fundus images analysis using deep features for detection of exudates, hemorrhages and microaneurysms. In: BMC Ophthalmology (2018)
4. Klein, S., Staring, M., Murphy, K., Viergever, M.A., Pluim, J.P.W.: elastix: a toolbox for intensity-based medical image registration. IEEE Trans. Med. Imag. **29**(1), 196–205 (2010). https://doi.org/10.1109/TMI.2009.2035616
5. Lam, C., Yi, D., Guo, M., Lindsey, T.: Automated detection of diabetic retinopathy using deep learning. AMIA Joint Summits on Translational Science proceedings. AMIA Joint Summits on Translational Science 2017, 147–155 (2018)
6. Li, Y., Gregori, G., Knighton, R.W., Lujan, B., Rosenfeld, P.: Registration of OCT fundus images with color fundus photographs based on blood vessel ridges. Opt. Express **19**, 7–16 (2011). https://doi.org/10.1364/OE.19.000007
7. Li, Z., Huang, F., Zhang, J., Dashtbozorg, B., Abbasi-Sureshjani, S., Sun, Y., Long, X., Yu, Q., ter Haar Romeny, B., Tan, T.: Multi-modal and multi-vendor retina image registration. Biomed. Opt. Express **9**(2), 410–422 (2018)
8. Liskowski, P., Krawiec, K.: Segmenting retinal blood vessels with deep neural networks. IEEE Trans. Med. Imag. **35**, 1–1 (2016)
9. Mattes, D., Haynor, D.R., Vesselle, H., Lewellyn, T.K., Eubank, W.: Nonrigid multimodality image registration. Proc. SPIE - Int. Soc. Opt. Eng. **4322**, 1609–1620 (2001). https://doi.org/10.1117/12.431046
10. Miri, M.S., Abramoff, M., Kwon, Y.H., Garvin, M.K.: Multimodal registration of SD-OCT volumes and fundus photographs using histograms of oriented gradients. Biomed. Opt. Express **7**, 5252–5267 (2016)
11. Novais, E., Baumal, C., Sarraf, D., Freund, K., Duker, J.: Multimodal imaging in retinal disease: a consensus definition. Ophthalmic Surg. Lasers & Imag. Retina **47**, 201–205 (2016). https://doi.org/10.3928/23258160-20160229-01
12. Otsu, N.: A threshold selection method from gray-level histograms. IEEE Trans. Syst. Man Cybern. **9**(1), 62–66 (1979)
13. Palén, A.: Advanced algorithms for manipulating 2D objects on touch screens. Master's thesis, Tampere University of Technology (2016)
14. Ronneberger, O., Fischer, P., Brox, T.: U-Net: convolutional networks for biomedical image segmentation. In: Navab, N., Hornegger, J., Wells, W.M., Frangi, A.F. (eds.) MICCAI 2015. LNCS, vol. 9351, pp. 234–241. Springer, Cham (2015). https://doi.org/10.1007/978-3-319-24574-4_28
15. Schlegl, T., et al.: Fully automated detection and quantification of macular fluid in OCT using deep learning. Ophthalmology **125**(4), 549–558 (2018)
16. Schmitz-Valckenberg, S., Holz, F., Bird, A., Spaide, R.F.: Fundus autofluorescence imaging: review and perspectives. Retina (Philadelphia, Pa.) **28**, 385–409 (2008). https://doi.org/10.1097/IAE.0b013e318164a907
17. Zana, F., Klein, J.C.: A multimodal registration algorithm of eye fundus images using vessels detection and hough transform. IEEE Trans. Med. Imag. **18**(5), 419–428 (1999). https://doi.org/10.1109/42.774169

Automated Enriched Medical Concept Generation for Chest X-ray Images

Aydan Gasimova$^{(\boxtimes)}$

Imperial College London, London, UK
`a.gasimova16@imperial.ac.uk`

Abstract. Decision support tools that rely on supervised learning require large amounts of expert annotations. Using past radiological reports obtained from hospital archiving systems has many advantages as training data above manual single-class labels: they are expert annotations available in large quantities, covering a population-representative variety of pathologies, and they provide additional context to pathology diagnoses, such as anatomical location and severity. Learning to auto-generate such reports from images present many challenges such as the difficulty in representing and generating long, unstructured textual information, accounting for spelling errors and repetition/redundancy, and the inconsistency across different annotators. We therefore propose to first learn visually-informative medical concepts from raw reports, and, using the concept predictions as image annotations, learn to auto-generate structured reports directly from images. We validate our approach on the OpenI [2] chest x-ray dataset, which consists of frontal and lateral views of chest x-ray images, their corresponding raw textual reports and manual medical subject heading (MeSH$^{®}$) annotations made by radiologists.

Keywords: NLP · Medical imaging · Deep learning

1 Introduction

Radiologists are faced daily with the very time-consuming and repetitive task of looking at hundreds of radiography images and writing up radiological reports. The fast turn-arounds they are expected to produce leads to fatigue that can negatively affect diagnostic accuracy [18]. Supervised learning for automated pathology detection from images has the potential for clinical-decision support, however, such image segmentation and classification learning tasks require detailed annotations covering a large distribution of input data for the algorithms to be able to make robust predictions. Such annotations must be made by qualified radiologists, which, for the detail and breadth of annotation required, will be an equally if not more time-consuming task than manually creating the reports. In addition, classification and semantic segmentation tasks only solve for the prediction of presence of pathologies, and not the generation of reports which contain additional information such as severity, location, and absence of pathologies.

© Springer Nature Switzerland AG 2019
K. Suzuki et al. (Eds.): ML-CDS 2019/IMIMIC 2019, LNCS 11797, pp. 83–92, 2019.
https://doi.org/10.1007/978-3-030-33850-3_10

Recently, we have seen supervised learning approaches that aim to take advantage of past radiological exams containing reports in order to either auto-generate the reports [9,16,22], or to assist in classification tasks [15,19–21,23]. The noise present in medical reports in addition to the presence of non-visually significant information, such as the negation of pathologies, make it difficult to learn from them directly as done in natural image captioning frameworks. Additionally, high recall/precision of pathologies is more crucial in the medical domain where the risk of mis-labelling is much higher.

We therefore propose to use a limited number of manual medical concept annotations in order to first learn to extract them from raw reports, and then take advantage of the model predictions as image annotations, thus providing a method for augmenting an image-annotation dataset. We then demonstrate how these image-concept annotations can be learned through sequence models conditioned on image features, and generate a more readable context for the diagnosis that can be used as part of a clinical decision support system, thus greatly alleviating the burden on radiologists. Our approach can be summarised in the following steps:

1. We propose a network that learns to extract visually-significant medical concepts from raw reports. To our knowledge, this is a first attempt to that goes beyond simple pathology detection to include concepts such as anatomical position and severity.
2. We explore several sequence-learning networks that aim to condition the sequence generation process on image features in order to learn to auto-generate structured reports from radiological images.
3. We use the predictions made by the structured report generation process in step 1 to demonstrate how they can be used to create an image-report training set for step 2.

2   Related Work

2.1   Data-Mining Image Labels

There are two common approaches to extracting image labels from raw reports: statistical and tool based. Radiological text mapping tools such as DNorm [12] and MetaMap [3] have been used to extract labels for multi-label classification [21] and in weakly supervised localisation learning frameworks [20]. However, other biological concepts in the reports, such as location, severity, and other visually descriptive features of the pathology are not taken advantage of. Unsupervised, statistical methods such as latent Dirichlet allocation [15] and clustering [19] have been used to implicitly define topics and cluster groups containing key words and propose classification into these topics and groups. These approaches are heavily dependent on the number of topics/groups providing the lowest perplexity score, which can be a range of values. In addition, these are not generative models, therefore reports can only be selected based on nearest-neighbour methods. To this end, we propose instead to learn to generate reports comprised of medical concept from images, in a similar style to natural image captioning.

2.2 Radiology Report Generation

Closest to our work, Shin et al. proposed a cascaded learning framework to auto-generate MeSH annotations from chest X-rays [16] whereby image embeddings are first extracted from a pre-trained classification network, and then used to initialise a sequence prediction model to auto-generate MeSH sequences. Zhang et al. [22,23] leverage manually created structured reports in a dual-attention framework to improve features used for classifying histopathology images and to provide interpretability to the classification. The reports used in both cases are far more structured than their raw counterparts and so this approach cannot be directly translated to hospital data. Training on raw hospital reports, Jing et al. [9] demonstrated how they can be generated by first training a multi-label CNN on the images and the Medical Text Indexer (MTI) tags identified in the original raw reports of the Openi chest x-ray dataset. However, reports can be very long and heterogeneous, and the authors do not evaluate the model's ability to determine whether visually and clinically-relevant medical concepts have been identified. To address the challenges of learning from raw reports directly, we first learn to generate structured reports made up of only visually-significant medical concepts that correspond directly to features seen in the images. Being shorter and vocabulary-controlled, the generation process is easier to evaluate for correct identification of pathologies.

3   Method

3.1   Enriched Concept Extraction from Raw Reports

We approach learning structured reports from raw textual reports as a multi-label classification task since the vocabulary of MeSH terms is consistent across annotators, and limited. We modify the shallow CNN first introduced by Kim [10] for multi-class text classification and later adapted for multi-label text classification by Liu et al. [13] by introducing a learn-able embedding layer as we do not have the advantage of pre-trained word embeddings for medical text, and by introducing dropout followed by a fully-connected layer to each convolutional output prior to the concatenation to aid regularisation.

Let $x_i \in \mathbb{R}^d$ be the d-dimensional word vector for the i-th word of report p. The textual report is thus represented as a concatenation of word embeddings: $p = [x_0, ...x_i, ...x_M] \in \mathbb{R}^{M \times d}$ where M is the maximum length of the reports. A filter $m \in \mathbb{R}^{hd}$ is convolved with a window of h words to produce a new feature c_i:

$$c_j = f(m * x_{i:i+h-1} + b) \tag{1}$$

where f is a non-linear activation function and b is a bias term. The filter is applied consecutively to every h-word window in the sentence, resulting in a feature map $c = [c_0, ...c_i, ...c_{M-h+1}] \in \mathbb{R}^{M-h+1}$. Max-over-time pooling [4] is applied over each feature map to capture the most important feature $\hat{c} = max(c)$. In this way we apply many filter operations with varying window widths in order to obtain multiple features that are able to capture semantic information of reports with varying word lengths. We use the sigmoid activation function as we require an independent prediction for each class and train by minimising the multi-class sigmoid cross-entropy (SCE) loss. In addition, we add terms to balance maximising the true positive class prediction with true negative class predictions as the positive label space is very sparse:

$$\widehat{SCE}_i = -\lambda_1 \sum_{j=1}^{K} (y_j log(f(s_{ij})) + (1 - y_j log(1 - f(s_j)))$$

$$- \lambda_2 \sum_{j=1}^{K} y_j f(s_j) / \sum_{j=1}^{K} (y_j f(s_j) + y_j(1 - f(s_j)))$$

$$- \lambda_3 \sum_{j=1}^{K}(1 - y_j)(1 - f(s_j)) / \sum_{j=1}^{K}((1 - y_j)(1 - f(s_j)) + (1 - y_j)(f(s_j)))$$

$$(2)$$

where K is the number of classes, y_j is presence/absence of class label j for instance i, $f(s_j)$ is the prediction for instance i on label j made through a sigmoid activation:

$$f(s_i) = \frac{1}{1 + e^{-s_i}} \tag{3}$$

The weights of each loss term, $\lambda_1, \lambda_2, \lambda_3$ are non-negative, sum to 1 and chosen through cross-validation. Finally, the modified SCE loss is averaged over batches.

3.2   Report Generation from Images

Given that it is possible to learn structured report outputs from raw reports, we propose a method of learning to auto-generate structured reports directly from images. We explore multiple ways of conditioning the MeSH sequence learning on the image embeddings that aims to maintain the dependency between the word generation process and the image embedding at every time-step. The MeSH sequence is modelled using an RNN, specifically the Long Short-Term Memory (LSTM) implementation proposed in [8]. Each LSTM unit has three sigmoid gates to control the internal state: 'input', 'output' and 'forget'. At each time step, the gates control how much of the previous time steps is propagated through to determine the output. For an input word sequence $\{x_1, \ldots, x_n\}$ where $x_i \in \mathbb{R}^d$, the internal hidden state $h_t \in \mathbb{R}^h$ and memory state $m_t \in \mathbb{R}^m$ are updated as follows:

$$h_t = f_t \odot h_{t-1} + i_t \odot \tanh(W^{(hx)}x_t + W^{(hm)}m_{t-1})$$
$$m_t = o_t \odot \tanh(h_t) \tag{4}$$

where $x_t \in \mathbb{R}^D$ is the word embedding, $W^{(hx)}$ and $W^{(hm)}$ are the trainable weight parameters, and i_t, o_t and f_t are the input, output and forget gates respectively. Bias terms are left out for readability.

The image embedding, $\boldsymbol{im}_i = \text{CNN}(I)$ where $\boldsymbol{im}_i \in \mathbb{R}^g$ is extracted from the final spatial-average pooling layer of the pre-trained CNN. We explore three ways of conditioning the sequence learning process:

1. RNN0: The image embedding is projected into the same embedding space as the word embeddings via a dense transition layer: $\boldsymbol{im} = \text{relu}(W^{(dg)}\text{CNN}(I))$. The image embedding is concatenated with the word sequence and thus treated as the first 'word' in the MeSH sequence.
2. RNN1: The image embedding is projected via a dense transition layer into a fixed embedding width and combined with the output of the recurrent layer through either concatenation or summation operation, and passed to the decoder dec:

$$\boldsymbol{dec}_t = \text{relu}(W^{(z)}(o_t * \text{relu}(W^{(dg)}\text{CNN}(I)))) \tag{5}$$

where $*$ represents concatenation or summation and W^z are the weights of the decoder.
3. RNN2: The image embedding is projected via a dense transition layer into a fixed embedding width and combined with the input of the recurrent layer through either concatenation or summation operation, and passed to the encoder enc:

$$\boldsymbol{enc}_t = \text{relu}(W^{(a)}(x_t * \text{relu}(W^{(dg)}\text{CNN}(I)))) \tag{6}$$

where W^a are the weights of the encoder.

The model architectures are illustrated in Fig. 1. For all models, the decoder outputs are passed to the prediction layer $s(t) = f(W^T x_t)$ where f is the softmax function. The models are all trained by minimising the cross-entropy loss between the output and true sequence:

$$L(S, I) = -\sum_{t=0}^{T} \log p(P_t = T_t | \text{CNN}(I), P_0 \ldots P_{t-1}) \tag{7}$$

where p is the probability that the predicted word P_t equals the true word T_t at time step t given image features $\text{CNN}(I)$ and previous words $P_0 \ldots P_{t-1}$, and T is the LSTM sequence length.

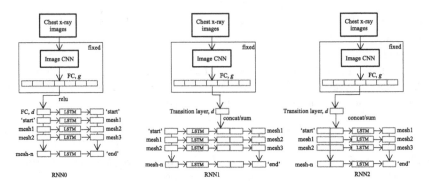

Fig. 1. Image-MeSH sequence learning model architectures.

4   Experiments

4.1   Dataset

We evaluated our models on the OpenI [2] Indiana U. Chest X-ray Collection. This dataset consists of 7,470 frontal and lateral chest x-ray images and 3,955 associated radiological reports from the hospital's picture archiving systems. They have all been fully anonymised to remove patient names. In addition to the raw text reports, each exam has MeSH annotations made by qualified radiologists. MeSH annotations are (with some exceptions) formatted as [pathology/description, ... pathology/description] where *description* is a combination of *anatomy/position/severity*. The number of captions per image is on average 2.33, with an average of 2.68 MeSH terms per caption.

Preprocessing. This involved lower-casing, punctuation and non-alphanumeric character removal from reports and MeSH. We limit the MeSH annotations to just one *pathology/description* pair by selecting the caption with the most common pathology. Additionally, as the negation of pathologies was generally standard across reports, we performed negation removal using regex. Finally, the text reports were cropped/padded to 32 words based on the average of $20.23 + 1$ std of 11.9. MeSH captions were cropped/padded to length 5 based on average $+ 1$ std. Empty reports were removed. This resulted in 3,023 unique report-MeSH term pairs, of which 300 were randomly selected for validation and 300 for test.

4.2   Experimental Settings

We first investigate whether the structured reports can be learned from raw reports by creating a sub-set of size $= 1000$ of the MeSH annotated reports, and training the text CNN on the report-MeSH pairs in the sub-set. The trained text CNN is then used to make MeSH prediction on the remaining set of raw reports, and these (together with the gold-standard annotated sub-set from the previous step) are used to train the image-MeSH sequence model. We compare this to training the image-MeSH sequence model on the entire gold-standard annotated set of 3,023.

Text CNN. For the text CNN model, we use rectified linear units as activation function on the convolutional layers, one-dimensional convolutional filters of width 3, 4, 5 with 512 feature maps for each filter, dropout rate [5] of p = 0.5, with 254 hidden units for the dense layer, and with $\lambda_1 = 0.5, \lambda_2 = 0.2, \lambda_3 = 0.3$ for the loss terms. The model was trained through batch backpropagation, batch size = 128 and using Adam optimisation [11] with learning rate = 0.001 for 100 epochs with early-stopping. To compensate for the class imbalance of 'normal' vs. diseased cases, we select batches with uniform distribution over the classes, augmenting the instances by sentence-shuffling.

Sequence Models. Image embeddings are extracted from the last average pooling layers of Vgg16 [17] and Resnet50 [7] models, pre-trained on ImageNet [6] to extract $im \in \mathbb{R}^{4096}$ and $im \in \mathbb{R}^{2048}$ respectively. For RNN0, the joint image-word embedding dim is set to 2048 for the Vgg input, and 1024 for Resnet. For RNN1 and RNN2, the dense transition layer dimension is set to 1024. For all the sequence models, the LSTM hidden state is set to dim 512, and the LSTM units are unrolled up to 6 time steps (1 for the start token, and 5 for MeSH sequence). All models are trained with batch size 128, using Adam optimisation [11], learning rate = 0.001 and early-stopping.

Table 1. Text CNN classification metrics for sub-sampled and full gold-standard annotated data. Metrics reported on test data.

All classes							
Training sample size	Acc.	R	R-OC	R-OS	P	P-OC	P-OS
1000	98.26	67.82	40.49	65.79	70.15	45.15	67.18
3023 (all)	99.48	92.07	84.50	91.77	89.90	84.82	89.47
Pathology classes							
Training sample	Acc.	R	R-OC	R-OS	P	P-OC	P-OS
1000	98.64	67.41	44.72	60.00	69.73	44.57	56.22
3023 (all)	99.54	90.74	86.94	80.67	88.45	86.35	78.72

5   Results

Enriched Concept Extraction from Reports. We evaluate the MeSH term prediction from the text reports by calculating the total binary accuracy (Acc),

Table 2. BLEU1–4 score comparisons on model in [16] and our RNN0, RNN1 and RNN2 trained on all gold-standard MeSH annotations, and trained on 1000 gold-standard MeSH annotations+textCNN predictions.

Model	Train	Val	Test
	B-1/B-2/B-3/B-4	B-1/B-2/B-3/B-4	B-1/B-2/B-3/B-4
Learning to read [16]	**97.2/67.1**/14.9/2.8	**68.1**/30.1/5.2/1.1	**79.3**/9.1/0.0/0.0
RNN0+vgg16+all	8.8/1.8/0.7/0.2	7.8/2.6/1.1/1.4	6.9/2.3/0.7/0.1
RNN0+resnet50+all	16.5/8.6/4.6/2.4	16.7/8.7/3.9/1.0	18.8/10.4/3.8/1.9
RNN1+resnet50+all	77.9/45.6/**29.4/18.9**	65.7/**51.6/30.2/17.1**	66.7/**47.1/26.8/15.9**
RNN2+resnet50+all	74.1/42.0/26.8/17.3	63.2/47.5/27.3/15.8	63.2/43.9/25.5/13.6
RNN0+resnet50+pred	22.9/15.5/7.8/4.0	13.6/8.3/4.0/0.9	14.7/9.3/2.7/1.5
RNN1+resnet50+pred	73.6/50.0/**30.9/17.8**	41.5/29.7/**15.9/7.2**	41.6/**28.2/13.2/8.1**
RNN2+resnet50+pred	69.4/47.6/29.6/16.7	39.4/28.0/14.6/6.7	39.8/26.4/12.7/8.0

precision (P) and recall (R), and the mean-over-class (P-OC, R-OC) and mean-over-samples (P-OS, R-OS) precision and recall of the 102 classes. In addition, we report metrics of the 'pathology' classes separately by manual allocation based on the definitions on the MeSH term online library [1]. Complete metrics are compared in Table 1.

Report Generation from Images. During inference, the first word is sampled from the LSTM, concatenated to the input, and used to predict consequent words. The quality of the generated reports was evaluated by measuring BLUE [14] scores averaged over all the reports, which are a form of n-gram precision commonly used for evaluating image captioning as they maintain high correlation with human judgement. BLEU scores of RNN0, RNN1 and RNN2 trained on all gold-standard annotations and on the predictions made by the text CNN are presented in Table 2. RNN0 is the same framework used in [16], however, they additionally train their model in a cascaded fashion which significantly improves the model's ability to predict the first word, but struggles to maintain visual correspondence in generating subsequent words, hence the steep reduction in higher n-gram precision. Additionally, cascaded models suffer from error propagation during test time, hence the poor performance on test data. RNN1 and RNN2 solve both problems by conditioning the word generation process on the images at every time-step and by being trained end-to-end, hence achieving higher n-gram scores on the test data. In addition, we have shown that we can achieve comparably high BLEU metrics when training on the predicted MeSH terms made by the text CNN.

6   Conclusion

We demonstrate how, given a small amount of manual annotations, clinically and visually-important concepts can be learned from raw textual radiology reports.

We then demonstrate how these concepts can be used as radiological image annotations and used in an image-sequence learning model to auto-generate reports as part of a clinical decision support system.

References

1. Medical subject headings - national library of medicine. https://meshb.nlm.nih. gov/
2. Open-i: An open access biomedical search engine. https://openi.nlm.nih.gov/
3. Aronson, A.R.: Effective mapping of biomedical text to the UMLs Metathesaurus: the MetaMap program. In: Proceedings of the AMIA Symposium, p. 17. American Medical Informatics Association (2001)
4. Collobert, R., Weston, J., Bottou, L., Karlen, M., Kavukcuoglu, K., Kuksa, P.: Natural language processing (almost) from scratch. J. Mach. Learn. Res. **12**, 2493–2537 (2011)
5. Dahl, G.E., Sainath, T.N., Hinton, G.E.: Improving deep neural networks for LVCSR using rectified linear units and dropout. In: 2013 IEEE International Conference on Acoustics, Speech and Signal Processing, pp. 8609–8613. IEEE (2013)
6. Deng, J., Dong, W., Socher, R., Li, L.J., Li, K., Fei-Fei, L.: ImageNet: a large-scale hierarchical image database. In: 2009 IEEE Conference on Computer Vision and Pattern Recognition, pp. 248–255. IEEE (2009)
7. He, K., Zhang, X., Ren, S., Sun, J.: Deep residual learning for image recognition. In: Proceedings of the IEEE Conference on Computer Vision and Pattern Recognition, pp. 770–778 (2016)
8. Hochreiter, S., Schmidhuber, J.: Long short-term memory. Neural Comput. **9**(8), 1735–1780 (1997)
9. Jing, B., Xie, P., Xing, E.: On the automatic generation of medical imaging reports. arXiv preprint arXiv:1711.08195 (2017)
10. Kim, Y.: Convolutional neural networks for sentence classification. arXiv preprint arXiv:1408.5882 (2014)
11. Kingma, D.P., Ba, J.: Adam: a method for stochastic optimization. arXiv preprint arXiv:1412.6980 (2014)
12. Leaman, R., Khare, R., Lu, Z.: Challenges in clinical natural language processing for automated disorder normalization. J. Biomed. Inform. **57**, 28–37 (2015)
13. Liu, J., Chang, W.C., Wu, Y., Yang, Y.: Deep learning for extreme multi-label text classification. In: Proceedings of the 40th International ACM SIGIR Conference on Research and Development in Information Retrieval, pp. 115–124. ACM (2017)
14. Papineni, K., Roukos, S., Ward, T., Zhu, W.J.: BLEU: a method for automatic evaluation of machine translation. In: Proceedings of the 40th Annual Meeting on Association for Computational Linguistics, pp. 311–318. Association for Computational Linguistics (2002)
15. Shin, H.C., Lu, L., Kim, L., Seff, A., Yao, J., Summers, R.M.: Interleaved text/image deep mining on a large-scale radiology database for automated image interpretation. J. Mach. Learn. Res. **17**(1–31), 2 (2016)
16. Shin, H.C., Roberts, K., Lu, L., Demner-Fushman, D., Yao, J., Summers, R.M.: Learning to read chest x-rays: recurrent neural cascade model for automated image annotation. In: Proceedings of the IEEE Conference on Computer Vision and Pattern Recognition, pp. 2497–2506 (2016)

17. Simonyan, K., Zisserman, A.: Very deep convolutional networks for large-scale image recognition. arXiv preprint arXiv:1409.1556 (2014)
18. Stec, N., Arje, D., Moody, A.R., Krupinski, E.A., Tyrrell, P.N.: A systematic review of fatigue in radiology: is it a problem? Am. J. Roentgenol. **210**(4), 799–806 (2018)
19. Wang, X., et al.: Unsupervised joint mining of deep features and image labels for large-scale radiology image categorization and scene recognition. In: 2017 IEEE Winter Conference on Applications of Computer Vision (WACV), pp. 998–1007. IEEE (2017)
20. Wang, X., Peng, Y., Lu, L., Lu, Z., Bagheri, M., Summers, R.M.: Chestx-ray8: hospital-scale chest x-ray database and benchmarks on weakly-supervised classification and localization of common thorax diseases. In: Proceedings of the IEEE Conference on Computer Vision and Pattern Recognition, pp. 2097–2106 (2017)
21. Yan, K., Peng, Y., Sandfort, V., Bagheri, M., Lu, Z., Summers, R.M.: Holistic and comprehensive annotation of clinically significant findings on diverse CT images: learning from radiology reports and label ontology. In: Proceedings of the IEEE Conference on Computer Vision and Pattern Recognition, pp. 8523–8532 (2019)
22. Zhang, Z., Chen, P., Sapkota, M., Yang, L.: TandemNet: distilling knowledge from medical images using diagnostic reports as optional semantic references. In: Descoteaux, M., Maier-Hein, L., Franz, A., Jannin, P., Collins, D.L., Duchesne, S. (eds.) MICCAI 2017. LNCS, vol. 10435, pp. 320–328. Springer, Cham (2017). https://doi.org/10.1007/978-3-319-66179-7_37
23. Zhang, Z., Xie, Y., Xing, F., McGough, M., Yang, L.: MDNet: a semantically and visually interpretable medical image diagnosis network. In: Proceedings of the IEEE Conference on Computer Vision and Pattern Recognition, pp. 6428–6436 (2017)

Correction to: Interpretability of Machine Intelligence in Medical Image Computing and Multimodal Learning for Clinical Decision Support

Kenji Suzuki, Mauricio Reyes, Tanveer Syeda-Mahmood,
Ender Konukoglu, Ben Glocker, Roland Wiest⦿, Yaniv Gur,
Hayit Greenspan, and Anant Madabhushi

Correction to:
K. Suzuki et al. (Eds.): *Interpretability of Machine Intelligence in Medical Image Computing and Multimodal Learning for Clinical Decision Support*, **LNCS 11797, https://doi.org/10.1007/978-3-030-33850-3**

The chapter titled "Incorporating Task-Specific Structural Knowledge into CNNs for Brain Midline Shift Detection" was revised. The names of two authors were spelled incorrectly and the grant number was missing the final digit. This was corrected.

The original version of this book was revised. Due to an error, the volume editor's affiliation "ETH Zurich" appeared on SpringerLink instead of his name "Ender Konukoglu." This was fixed.

The updated version of the book can be found at
https://doi.org/10.1007/978-3-030-33850-3_4
https://doi.org/10.1007/978-3-030-33850-3

© Springer Nature Switzerland AG 2020

K. Suzuki et al. (Eds.): ML-CDS 2019/IMIMIC 2019, LNCS 11797, p. C1, 2020.
https://doi.org/10.1007/978-3-030-33850-3_11

Author Index

Printed in the United States
By Bookmasters